Handbook of
Nitrous Oxide
and
Oxygen Sedation

D0834602

Handbook of

Nitrous Oxide
and
Oxygen Sedation

Morris S. Clark, DDS, FACD
Associate Professor and
Director of Anesthesia and Pain Control
Division of Oral and Maxillofacial Surgery
School of Dentistry
Associate Professor, Department of Otolaryngology
School of Medicine
University of Colorado
Denver, Colorado

Ann L. Brunick, RDH, MS
Chairperson and Associate Professor
Department of Dental Hygiene
University of South Dakota
Vermillion, South Dakota

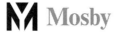

An Imprint of Elsevier Science

St. Louis   London   Philadelphia   Sydney   Toronto

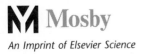

Mosby

An Imprint of Elsevier Science

Printed in the United States of America

Mosby, Inc.
11830 Westline Industrial Drive
St. Louis, MO 63146

ISBN 0-8151-8393-3

To Maureen, Gregory, and Angela,
the core of my life.
MSC

To Dr. Richard T. Ford,
a wonderful mentor from the beginning
ALB

⌗ Foreword

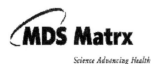

Science Advancing Health

MDS Matrx Medical is pleased that a text on the important subject of nitrous oxide/oxygen sedation has been undertaken. While MDS Matrx Medical provides state-of-the-art equipment for the delivery of these gases, a compendium of all facets pertinent to administration was needed. This book satisfies this need.

Patient management, particularly in the management of pain, must be accomplished with safety and compassion. As new information becomes available it must be added to the core understanding, thereby enhancing the subject matter.

This well-documented review touches on all the "hot buttons" with an openness that heretofore has been overlooked. It is written in a clear and concise format and undoubtedly ranks among the best texts of nitrous oxide/oxygen sedation to date. Texts of this stature serve to promote the safe use and understanding of this valuable modality of pain management.

Education is the key to knowledge.

Paul A. Baczkowski

Paul Baczkowski
Director of Engineering
MDS Matrx Medical

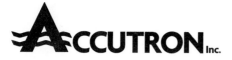

ACCUTRON_{Inc.}

When Dr. Clark and Ms. Brunick asked Accutron to prepare an acknowledgement for their new book, we were honored, but more importantly, we were impressed.

What impressed us most was the vision these two gifted professionals had in bringing the various disciplines of the nitrous oxide/oxygen sedation delivery community together during the research and review stages of the book.

Key elements for the successful practice of nitrous oxide/oxygen sedation are the practition-ers, educators, manufacturers of the nitrous oxide and oxygen gases, and the manufacturers of the gas delivery equipment. Each of these segments is necessary for delivery of nitrous oxide/oxygen sedation and each is identified in this book.

Bringing together all of the resources required tremendous energy, skilled diplomacy, and a never-ending pursuit of excellence. This book demonstrates that Dr. Clark and Ms. Brunick always exceeded in meeting these goals while never forgetting that patient safety and good science are paramount.

All of us at Accutron are very excited about this book and its clear, concise method of pro-viding the most vital N_2O/O_2 sedation information necessary for every professional in the medical and dental community.

Nitrous oxide/oxygen sedation has a 150-year history of safe and effective treatment of patient fear and anxiety. We at Accutron are all very proud to be a part of providing this incredible tool that makes medical and dental treatment more productive and comfortable.

This book is a valuable addition to the world of nitrous oxide/oxygen sedation.

Congratulations on a job well done.

James Moore
Vice President
Accutron, Inc.
Phoenix, Arizona

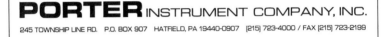

PORTER INSTRUMENT COMPANY, INC.

245 TOWNSHIP LINE RD.   P.O. BOX 907   HATFIELD, PA 19440-0907   (215) 723-4000 / FAX (215) 723-2199

In this book, Dr. Morris Clark and Ms. Ann Brunick continue the noble service of demystifying the concepts and utilization of nitrous oxide/oxygen conscious sedation. Having celebrated its 150th anniversary in 1994, nitrous oxide has clearly established an impressive safety record while providing practitioners an important tool to deal with the anxiety and pain control of their patients. Porter Instrument is proud to be part of this collaborative effort and will continue to develop products that will meet the needs of practitioners and patients in the future.

Gary Porter
Porter Instrument Company, Inc.
Hatfield, Pennsylvania

⌗ About the Book

This book was intentionally designed to provide a fresh, visual, updated text on nitrous oxide/oxygen sedation. We felt it should be adaptable to any health discipline whether practitioners were using it for the first time or have been using it and need a refresher.

We have done an extensive literature review on all aspects of this and related topics. However, there is no doubt that our bibliographies are noninclusive. We commend all researchers and authors who have explored various aspects of this subject. We encourage you to seek additional information as you need it; our references will get you started. Please feel free to photocopy the appendices for use in your clinical settings.

The purpose of the format was to provide information in a quick, ready, reference form that would be user-friendly. It was meant to be brief and devoid of extraneous verbiage. It was designed to provide an adequate number of illustrations and photographs for you, the visually-oriented reader. Hopefully, the handbook size will facilitate your reference needs in the clinical setting. It is our intention for this to be an affordable and practical reference for students, residents, educators, and practitioners.

We believe we have provided a concise, comprehensive resource without sacrifice of information or respect for the subject. We welcome any comments for future revisions.

Preface

Many thoughts and emotions preceded the decision to write a text on nitrous oxide/oxygen sedation. After careful reflection, two concepts emerged—*enthusiasm* and *faith*.

Since its discovery, nitrous oxide has fascinated humankind. After more than 150 years of continuous use, it is still the most widely used anesthetic gas in the world today. Nitrous oxide was first observed in a sideshow performance by the dentist, Horace Wells. He immediately adapted its recreational use into a short-term anesthetic deemed appropriate for dentistry. Until his death he invested his finances, professional reputation, and his body for self-experimentation to expose the virtues of nitrous oxide as a significant agent in the humane treatment of patients—*enthusiasm-faith*.

I was invited to speak to the faculty and students at the University of South Dakota Department of Dental Hygiene. This course was supported by a grant written and procured by my coauthor, Ms. Ann Brunick, for the purpose of introducing nitrous oxide/oxygen sedation into the curriculum. Bringing this topic into the department not only educated students on this newly delegated duty for hygienists in the state, but also provided a safe, effective, time-proven method of comfort for their clinic patients—*enthusiasm-faith*.

This book is written with passion, and hopefully, sensitivity for application into any clinical setting that will benefit both patient and practitioner regardless of medical specialty or discipline. We have drawn on the tremendous strength from the *enthusiasm* and *faith* that has been clinically demonstrated by the increasing number of practitioners in health professions from podiatry to endoscopy, dentistry to dermatology. We hope this book will be valuable in your clinics and operatories, and that you will find it a useful reference to administer nitrous oxide/oxygen sedation enthusiastically!

Morris S. Clark

Dr. Clark was procured through a University grant to educate the faculty and students at the University of South Dakota Department of Dental Hygiene on the newly delegated function of nitrous oxide/oxygen administration and monitoring. As he and I were perusing the course evaluations, it became apparent that the participants were not completely satisfied with the reference texts currently available. It was then that I saw the *enthusiasm* to which Dr. Clark has referred. It was time to begin writing the book he had always wanted to write. He possesses an innate compassion for the comfort and well-being of all people. He feels strongly about spreading the word *enthusiastically* that nitrous oxide/oxygen is a viable treatment modality.

His reference to *faith* is clear. Dr. Clark *believes* that in today's world of ambulatory care, the option of using nitrous oxide/oxygen sedation should be a primary consideration. Dr. Clark *believes* nitrous oxide/oxygen therapy can serve many facets in the health professions and he *believes* the majority of patients' negative experiences with nitrous oxide have been caused by an inappropriate administration technique. Patients who think the drug made them feel worse rather than better were, most likely, oversedated by the practitioner. Dr. Clark has *faith* in this treatment modality, *faith* in your competency, and *faith* that you will find its use beneficial.

As for me, maybe Dr. Clark could sense my work ethic and inherent nature to do my best for students and patients. Maybe I was in the right place at the right time. I believe there are many of you who should have been his coauthor, but because of his *faith* in me, I have had the opportunity of a lifetime.

Ann L. Brunick

⌗ Acknowledgments

We would like to acknowledge all of the healthcare practitioners, too numerous to mention, who have dedicated their lives to pursuing excellence in patient care and who strive toward that highest, noble calling of alleviating pain and anxiety in our fellow humans.

We would especially like to thank those individuals who were instrumental in assisting us in various ways throughout the process of writing this book. First of all, we would like to thank the three equipment manufacturers in the United States who funded our way to visit their companies and warmly welcomed us during our stay. We were impressed at the collegiality among them. It is obvious that they want to produce quality equipment that ensures the safe delivery of nitrous oxide/oxygen around the world. Each of them contributed financially to the fulfillment of this project; their support is greatly appreciated. To begin, and listed in order of visitation, we would like to gratefully acknowledge Mr. Jim Moore at Accutron, Inc. for his hospitality and applaud him for his sincere interest in academic research. Further, our heartfelt appreciation goes to Mr. Gary Porter and Mr. Mike Lynam of Porter Instrument Co. Inc., for their generous hospitality and impressive discussion of the evolution of their unique products. We would also like to sincerely thank Mr. Dan Horrigan, Mr. Paul Baczkowski, Mr. Bill Hogan, and Mr. Neal Murray at MDS Matrx Medical Co., for their gracious hospitality, an insightful presentation regarding the international community, and futuristic vision of nitrous oxide/oxygen delivery. We hold our positive relationship with these companies and individuals in high regard.

We are grateful to David Swedlow, MD at Nellcor Puritan Bennett Inc., San Francisco, for introducing us to the manufacturing aspects of nitrous oxide. Dr. Swedlow facilitated our meeting Mr. Bill Fettes at the Nellcor Puritan Bennett, Inc. facility in Overland Park, KS. Mr. Fettes has been a terrific resource for us and a tremendous supporter of our project. We sincerely thank him for his expertise and willingness to assist us with the draft manuscript.

Special thanks to all those at the University of South Dakota Lommen Health Science Library, Mrs. Pat Hubert at the USD Educational Media Center, Mr. Simon Spicer at USD Photographic Services, Ms. DeAnna Miller, Ms. Bev Murra, Ms. Audrey Ticknor, and Mr. Travis Fisher for their assistance.

Several individuals deserve thanks from the University of Colorado Health Sciences Center for providing assistance with this project; special thanks are extended to Dr. Donald Kleier and Dr. Jim Lindenmuth. In addition, thank you to Mr. Kevin Clark, Mr. Matthew DeBenedictis, Mr. Raymond Clark, Dr. William Limongelli, Mr. Peter Ferucci, Dr. Clyde McDowell, Dr. Theodore Borden, and Dr. Milt Jaffe.

Special acknowledgment goes to Dr. Pete Jacobsohn for his untiring dedication to the honor of Horace Wells. We thank him for his contribution of historical materials for this book.

We were very fortunate to be able to include invaluable comments and suggestions from Mr. Ira Wainless, Senior Industrial Hygienist at the U.S. Department of Labor/OSHA.

Lastly, our heartfelt appreciation goes to Angela Reiner at Mosby, Inc., for her dedication and care, to Ms. Holly Roseman for her expertise, and to Ms. Linda Duncan and Ms. Penny Rudolph for their confidence in us and this project and for their personal and professional advice as editors at Mosby, Inc.

Contents

Introduction to Nitrous Oxide/Oxygen Sedation

Since its discovery 150 years ago nitrous oxide (N_2O) has been used to provide pain and anxiety relief to patients undergoing surgical procedures. More than 24 million surgical cases are performed each year in the United States,[1] and in most of them nitrous oxide/oxygen (N_2O/O_2) in combination with other drugs is used for general anesthesia. In addition to its use as a general anesthetic adjuvant, myriad health disciplines use N_2O/O_2 sedation as an effective means of alleviating patient anxiety and mild discomfort during ambulatory and outpatient procedures. For the patient, N_2O/O_2 provides pain control and anxiety relief that is quickly and easily reversed without unwanted side effects. For the practitioner the drug is easily titrated to the level required for the procedure while accommodating the patient's physiologic and psychologic needs.

N_2O has been cited extensively in the literature for 150 years as a safe and effective drug, and most of the early literature refers to dentistry as the discipline that first acknowledged its anesthetic potential. N_2O is notable because of its impeccable safety record. It has withstood the test of time longer than any other drug. Gardner Quincy Colton (1864 to 1897), an itinerant professor, documented 193,000 cases with no adverse reactions.[2] Ruben,[3] a Danish researcher, cites 3,000,000 cases using N_2O/O_2 in the dental office with no adverse reactions noted. Niels Bjorn Jorgensen[4] attests that 4,000,000 episodes without complications occurred in Denmark since 1956.

When used as a mild analgesic and sedative, N_2O is administered with oxygen from safe equipment that allows no more than 70% nitrous oxide and no less than 30% oxygen to be delivered at any time. The patient is awake and fully conscious and always able to respond to the direction of the practitioner. Protective defenses such as the cough and gag reflexes remain intact; clinical action and elimination are rapid. After a minimum postoperative oxygenation period of 3 to 5 minutes, the patient is recovered. There are no serious side effects associated with N_2O, provided the operator is using updated equipment and appropriate technique. Most often, persons who have had negative experiences with N_2O have been oversedated by the operator. To that end, this text will emphasize the titration aspect of the administration technique.

Because this text focuses on the use of nitrous oxide/oxygen in an ambulatory setting, which uses N_2O/O_2 for only minimal periods, we concur with others that adverse effects are negligible when treating the average, healthy patient, though certain circumstances may require postponement of N_2O/O_2 use. Of greater importance, however, are the effects of continual N_2O exposure to the healthcare professional. Previous research, whether valid, flawed, retrospective, or sound, has concerned many practitioners to the point that some have discontinued the use of N_2O/O_2. However, primarily because of the knowledge and attention of equipment manufacturers, methods of scavenging or minimizing trace gas have been incorporated to the extent that those in the healthcare industry can feel comfortable and confident about delivering N_2O/O_2 sedation without worry about their health. Conscientious clinicians will use recommended scavenging techniques as well as methods for minimizing trace gas contamination to provide a safe workplace for those exposed to N_2O.

We have seen many changes during our tenure as healthcare professionals. New drugs and diseases have revolutionized the way we practice. We practice with universal precautions. We use the latest technology. We adapt; we change. Sometimes we believe, sometimes we relent, and often we are regulated. Using appropriate N_2O/O_2 administration techniques and following recommended procedures for scavenging trace gas are no different than routinely wearing gloves.

N_2O/O_2 sedation may not provide the desired results for all patients, nor will it be an option for all practitioners; however, we invite you to take a new look at the subject. We suggest you trust the manufacturers' updated equipment, practice the administration technique described in this text, and follow the recommendations for minimizing trace gas contamination. N_2O/O_2 sedation is safe, easy to use, and effective for many clinical situations.

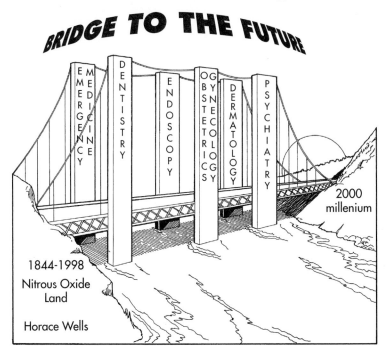

REFERENCES

1. Kole T: Assessing the potential for awareness and learning under anesthesia, *J Am Assoc of Nurse Anes* 61:571-577, 1993.
2. Chancellor JW: Dr. Wells' impact on dentistry and medicine, *J Am Dent Assoc* 125:1585-1589, 1994.
3. Ruben H: Nitrous oxide analgesia in dentistry, *Br Dent J* 132:195-196, 1972.
4. Jorgensen NB: *Sedation, local and general anesthesia in dentistry,* ed 2, Philadelphia, 1985, Lea & Febiger.

Pain and Anxiety Management

Millions of people postpone or avoid medical/dental treatment because of the pain and anxiety associated with seeking health-care treatment. The thought of diagnostic testing is often enough to prevent individuals from even making an appointment. People will endure severe pain before seeking professional care. Pain is the primary complaint of approximately one half of the total number of persons seeking medical care.[1] Annually in the United States 155 million people are in acute pain at least once during the year,[1] and statistics show that as many as 35 million people in the United States avoid the dental office because of their fear.[2] Often individuals find themselves in an emergency-room setting facing significant problems as a result of not having sought treatment at an earlier, more opportune time.

Managing a patient's pain and anxiety before performing a medical procedure provides an optimal environment with benefits to both patient and clinician. Obviously, if you the clinician know that your patient is relaxed and comfortable, you can provide better service with less stress (Figure 2-1). There are many options currently available for pain/anxiety relief. Some options in certain situations will prove more advantageous than others. But for many procedures several methods could be used. In those cases in which mild-to-moderate analgesia is needed and/or anxiety assistance would be beneficial, inhalation sedation using nitrous oxide/oxygen (N_2O/O_2) should be a primary consideration.

I. Mechanism of Pain

A. Definitions

Pain: As defined by the International Association for the Study of Pain: "an unpleasant sensory and emotional experience arising from actual or potential tissue damage. The experience includes

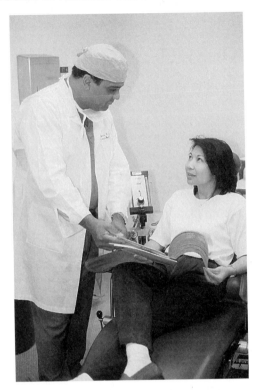

Figure 2-1   Reassuring the patient before surgery.

the perception of an uncomfortable stimulus and the response to that perception."[1]

B. Principles of action

   1. The objective of pain is to provide damage protection to tissue by alerting the central nervous system (CNS) before or during a potentially damaging occurrence.

      a. Pain receptors (nociceptors) are the first to receive a stimulus. These receptors are nonspecialized, bare nerve endings that record the occurrence, intensity, duration, and location of the sensation.[3]

      b. Impulses travel from the receptors along myelinated A-delta fibers and unmyelinated C fibers to the dorsal horn of the spinal cord. A-delta fibers are large and promote rapid conduction, whereas C fibers are smaller and carry impulses at a much slower rate.[3]

      c. It is at the dorsal horn of the spinal cord that the infamous gate control theory proposed by Melzack and Wall[4] functions. At the spinal cord a neurotransmitter called *substance P* is released, sending signals up the spinal tracts to the thalamus, the somatosensory portion of the cerebral cortex, and the reticular formation.[3]

d. Historically this process was thought to be the physiologic mechanism for transmitting impulses to the CNS, which would interpret and react to impulses. However, the current theory of pain modulation suggests that impulses are altered along the way by an endogenous opioid system. This concept promotes the fact that pain perception and reaction are organic components of the entire process.[5]

2. Modulation of pain impulses occurs through descending pathways stemming from the brain down to the spinal cord.

a. When the periaqueductal gray matter and the reticular formation are stimulated, the release of substance P is inhibited, preventing the pain impulse from being transmitted to the brain.

b. This endogenous analgesic system relies on built-in opiate neurotransmitters, which bind with opiate receptors at the terminal site of afferent fibers. Substance P cannot be released, thereby inhibiting the promulgation of the pain impulse (Figure 2-2).

3. Endogenous endorphins, enkephalins, and dynorphins have been discovered as substances that bind to the opiate receptors, resulting in pain modulation.[3,6] Activation of the endogenous opioid system can be accomplished by pain and/or stress.[7] Research of the endogenous opioid system continues.

4. Exogenous morphine also binds to an opiate receptor, which accounts for its analgesic properties. Morphine is the drug to which endogenous opiates and other opioid drugs are compared. Certain drugs are considered to be antagonists to opioid drugs. Naloxone hydrochloride (Narcan) will reverse the effects of opioid drugs and is most commonly used in acute overdose situations.[8]

5. Research has attempted to determine the role of N_2O on the endogenous opioid system. Gillman[9] proposes that analgesic concentrations of N_2O may act directly on the opioid receptor and/or activate the release of endogenous opiates.

6. Often, pain incites involuntary motor reflex action before the brain's acknowledgment of the impulse. This is the withdrawal reflex that separates body tissue from the noxious stimulus.

7. Reactions to pain vary from individual to individual and can vary from day to day. Several factors can influence pain reactions. Examples of these factors may be categorized as physical, mental, biochemical, psychologic, social, physiologic, cultural, and emotional.[1]

C. Assessing and measuring pain

1. Because of the wide variability among individuals regarding pain response, there is subjectivity involved in its interpretation by others. It is difficult to accurately interpret what each individual patient is feeling.

2. Healthcare professionals have made concerted efforts at identifying and quantifying the presence of pain. There

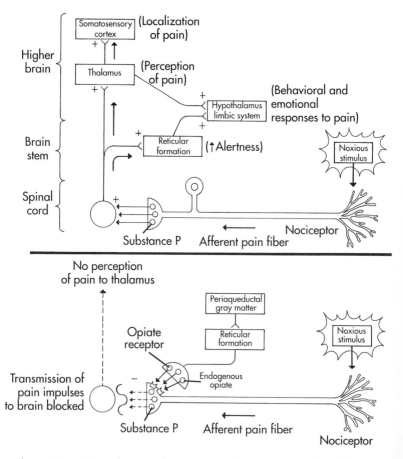

Figure 2-2   Pain pathway and proposed analgesic pathway. (Modified from Sherwood L: *Human physiology from cells to systems,* ed 2, 1993, Wadsworth Publishing Co.)

are a variety of scales intended to objectify the levels of pain in order to act appropriately and alleviate discomfort.[10-12] In many cases the scales have been helpful; however, some have not been useful.

a. Over the years many attempts have been made to objectify pain through numeric scales. A common scale depicts pain from 1 (very mild) to 10 (unbearable). Several other measures have been used; versions of various scales depict a range of happy to sad faces (Figure 2-3) for visually oriented populations such as children. Numeric scales prove useful when treating chronic pain because they serve as baseline references over time.

b. Even the simplest attempt to convey understanding of a patient's pain is admirable. For example, try using a word for pain from the patient's native language. Some examples are listed in Box 2-1.

c. Asking the patient about the extent of his/her pain communicates empathy toward the individual. Empathy is best expressed through direct eye contact. Problems

---

BOX 2-1
Words to Describe Pain in Other Languages

Dolor.......	Spanish	Aloum.........	Arabic
Itami.........	Japanese	Ponai..........	Greek
Tong.........	Chinese	Kú-av..........	Hebrew
Dau.........	Vietnamese	Tut weh.......	Yiddish
Douleur...	French	Wicayazan...	Lakota (Native American)
Bolit.........	Russian	Schmerz......	German
Pain.........	English		

0	1	2	3	4	5

Figure 2-3   Visual and numeric pain intensity scales. (From Wong: *Whaley & Wong's essentials of pediatric nursing,* ed 5, 1997, St Louis, Mosby.)

occur when healthcare professionals are presumptuous about how a patient should or should not feel. Any statement to a patient regarding how you think he/she feels will almost always be inaccurate, thereby exaggerating their discomfort level.

3. Healthcare professionals rely on continuing education and clinical experiences to guide them toward successful patient management. Inherent in this process is the ability to adapt and change to specific conditions. This process is dynamic and continuous; each experience develops better decision-making skills for the future and an intuitiveness, which is suppressed knowledge representing the sum quantity of all experiences encompassing both objective and subjective signs and symptoms. This sense aids in making rapid, rational, and reasonably accurate decisions, which frees the patient from pain and/or fear. Healthcare professionals gain confidence with successful decisions.

II. Mechanism of Fear/Anxiety

A. Definitions

1. Anxiety: *"A nonspecific feeling of apprehension, worry, uneasiness, or dread, the source of which may be vague or unknown. A normal reaction when one's body, lifestyle, values, or loved ones are threatened."[1]*

2. Fear: *"A feeling of fright or dread related to an identifiable source recognized by the individual."[1]*

3. Phobia: *"Any persistent and irrational fear of something specific, such as an object, activity, or situation that results in avoidance or desire to avoid the feared stimulus."[1]*

B. Interaction between fear and pain

1. Fear and pain are so interrelated that they are often hard to separate. Both have physiologic and emotional components.[13] As pain increases, anxiety is heightened; as anxiety increases, pain becomes enhanced and therefore less tolerable.[3] In a medical setting children cite fear of pain to be a significant obstacle.[14] When fear or pain is an issue, we ultimately manage both.

C. Assessing and measuring fear/anxiety

1. Objectively quantifying a patient's fear or anxiety poses a dilemma similar to pain. The greatest aspect of being human is individuality; however, because of our individ-

uality it is often difficult to make generalizations. There are several methods of assessing fear. Physiologic and behavioral signs often are overt indicators of fear. (White knuckle syndrome is depicted in Figure 2-4.) Self-reporting is becoming an accepted practice. A simple interview with a patient will uncover otherwise unspoken concerns. Similar to scales used with pain, there are many measurement devices that indicate fear and anxiety. The literature overflows with suggested indicators.[15-17] Obviously, crying, clinging, sweating, syncope, refusal to cooperate, silence, and obsessive talking are easily interpreted. Do not forget to consider chronic tardiness or last-minute appointment cancellations as anxiety related.

2. Repeatedly, we hear of patients carrying fear into their adult lives precipitating from a negative childhood experience in a medical or dental setting. Often patients have preconceived expectations of pain stemming from attitudes and behaviors displayed by parents, siblings,

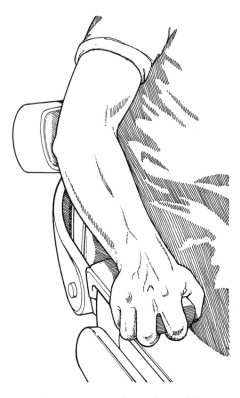

Figure 2-4 Words can be visible.

significant others, etc.[14] For those patients presenting with significant fear or even phobias, referral to an appropriate professional (i.e., child psychologist, etc.) is suggested. There are many management options available for these individuals.[18] It is crucial that every effort be made to ensure a positive experience for each patient.

D. Acknowledgment of fear/anxiety

1. When people indicate that they are anxious or fearful about something specific, they are expressing very intimate thoughts and placing themselves in a vulnerable position. It is an act of courage to openly express themselves while possibly becoming the subject of ridicule and judgment. Your appropriate acknowledgment solidifies their confidence in you and allows for an informed review of potential management options specific to every individual. This is a mutually beneficial situation as the patient claims ownership of his/her part in the treatment success while you enjoy reduced stress from a potentially complicated appointment.

2. Many of us have the ability to display sincere empathy to a patient. Empathy, which is best expressed through eye contact, has been cited as the greatest attribute a healthcare professional can possess.[19] By disclosing a genuine caring attitude, kindness, and concern for patients, we accomplish much more than our counterparts who do not possess these traits or cannot effectively communicate them. Patients do not have the ability to evaluate technical skills; therefore we are often judged by our communication skills. Those of us who are able to perform technical skills superiorly and provide treatment in a genuine, compassionate manner are truly blessed. We are the people to whom our patients refer others. Patients do not care what we know until they know that we care.

III. *Analgesia and Anesthesia*

A. Definitions

1. Analgesia:	*"Absence of a normal sense of pain"[1]*
2. Anesthesia:	*"Partial or complete loss of sensation, with or without loss of consciousness"[1]*
3. Sedation:	*"The process of allaying nervous excitement; the state of being calmed"[1]*

4. Conscious sedation: *"A minimally depressed level of consciousness during which the patient retains the ability to maintain a patent airway and respond appropriately to physical or verbal commands. This is accomplished by the use of appropriate analgesics and sedatives"*[1]

B. General anesthetic agents act as CNS depressants. Physiologists claim no consensus regarding the complete comprehensive understanding of the actual CNS or cellular site of action or molecular mechanism.[20] Accepted physiologic effects of these drugs include analgesia, amnesia, decreased reflex activity, skeletal muscle relaxation, and altered levels of consciousness.

C. Historically the process of inducing anesthesia and its accompanying physiologic manifestations has been studied by several professionals (i.e., Snow, Guedel, Gillespie).[21-23] Each observed various signs and symptoms and identified changes in stages of anesthetic progression. Many of these early findings are still used as benchmarks for observation of progressive increments of anesthesia today. Different resources identify slight variations of the titles and parameters of each stage; however, in general most professionals recognize four stages, which are listed in Box 2-2.

1. Stage I—Analgesia/Sedation represents patient responses from the initial action of the drug to the point when the person is in a relaxed and comfortable state. The patient is conscious and able to understand and follow verbal commands; pain is diminished to varying extents; fear/anxiety is reduced; and occasionally an altered perception of time may occur. It is critical to maintain constant observation of the patient so as not to overlook or miss any of the occurrences that signal the patient is moving into the next

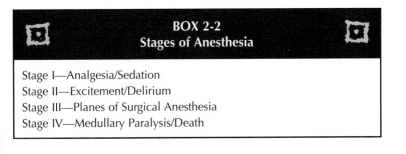

BOX 2-2
Stages of Anesthesia

Stage I—Analgesia/Sedation
Stage II—Excitement/Delirium
Stage III—Planes of Surgical Anesthesia
Stage IV—Medullary Paralysis/Death

stage. Stage I is the desired outcome when administering N₂O/O₂ sedation.

2. As CNS depression deepens, the patient enters Stage II—Excitement/Delirium. Often patients become combative and overreactive; their movements may become jerky and rigid. Be aware of subtle negative comments that directly or indirectly indicate a change in attitude. The patient will no longer appear as relaxed and comfortable as in Stage I. Stage II is quickly passed through when administering general anesthesia in a hospital setting. Patients undergoing N₂O/O₂ sedation in an ambulatory setting are frequently allowed to progress to this stage because of inadequate observation and/or inappropriate technique by the operator. Most often, the negative experiences associated with N₂O as expressed by the patient are the result of unrecognized progression into Stage II.

3. Major surgical procedures are most commonly performed in Stage III. The patient is unconscious and unable to breathe independently. In addition, laryngeal and pharyngeal reflexes are inactive. Three sublevels (planes) have been identified in this level, which further delineate the physiologic changes as one progresses through Stage III. With N₂O/O₂ it is difficult to reach the appropriate plane for performing a surgical procedure; however, it is possible to render a patient unconscious using N₂O/O₂.

4. If CNS depression continues, the planes of Stage III are quickly passed through and Stage IV—Medullary Paralysis/Death—results. In this stage respiratory arrest is followed by cardiac arrest. Clinical death may be reversed when the anesthetic agent is lessened and advanced life support measures are immediately used. This stage is extremely difficult to attain using N₂O/O₂.

IV. Spectrum of Pain and Anxiety Management Options

A. Several options are available for managing a patient's pain and anxiety. The spectrum begins with no intervention and ends with general anesthesia as an alternative (Figure 2-5). There are methods that use pharmacologic agents and others that do not. Options for consideration will be discussed

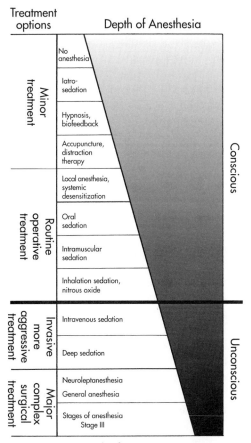

Treatment
options   Depth of Anesthesia

Minor treatment		No anesthesia
		Iatro-sedation
		Hypnosis, biofeedback
		Accupuncture, distraction therapy
Routine operative treatment		Local anesthesia, systemic desensitization
		Oral sedation
		Intramuscular sedation
		Inhalation sedation, nitrous oxide
Invasive more aggressive treatment		Intravenous sedation
		Deep sedation
Major complex surgical treatment		Neuroleptanesthesia / General anesthesia
		Stages of anesthesia Stage III

Conscious

Unconscious

Depth of Treatment

Figure 2-5   Pain and anxiety management options.

briefly. For additional information regarding any of these, several reputable texts and other resources are available.

1. Noninvasive, nonpharmacologic treatment procedures
   a. Iatrosedation may be defined as words and actions used by a clinician to facilitate a trusting relationship and positive rapport with a patient. This conscious choice of verbal and nonverbal communication is a vital component of every patient/operator interaction.[24] Positive attitudes, welcoming smiles, and a genuine display of kindness and concern reassure patients and may be all that is necessary to allay fear and anxiety. Iatrosedative language and actions are calm, slow, relaxing, and gentle.[25] Most often iatrosedation

is used to facilitate the effectiveness of other pharmacologic modalities.

b. Hypnosis is another nonpharmacologic method of providing pain and anxiety relief. Promoters suggest that hypnosis makes use of an individual's natural abilities.[26] Further study and training are necessary before using these techniques. Not everyone is hypnosuggestable; therefore this option is not reliable and does not enjoy widespread support.

c. Acupuncture and acupressure are similar to hypnosis in that they require further education and training before they are used. Their disadvantage, similar to hypnosis, is unreliability.

d. Systematic desensitization, relaxation therapy, biofeedback, distraction, and other coping strategies may be used to manage patient fear and anxiety. With the exception of distraction, these methods usually require the assistance of specialized professionals. Many resources are available that provide such services and/or information. Distraction mechanisms are intended to divert the individual's attention away from a fear-provoking stimulus. Examples of such distractions are reading materials in reception areas, music via office speakers or headphones, television, movies, aromatherapy, virtual reality headsets, and even manicures during dental procedures!

e. Transcutaneous electrical nerve stimulation (TENS) and electronic dental anesthesia (EDA) are pain-relieving methods that use electricity to prevent impulses from reaching the brain. Large A-fibers are stimulated electrically until the patient signals a tolerable twitching sensation. According to the Melzack and Wall[4] gate theory, impulses will not be propagated further, thus reducing pain. TENS also acts with the endogenous opioid system to produce endorphins and enkephalins.[27] Historically TENS has been used in physical therapy; however, dentistry has given TENS and EDA more exposure. The first and only blind, controlled study of TENS effectiveness was done by the author.[28] Several other studies indicate significant analgesic effects.[29-31]

2. Invasive, pharmacologic treatment procedures

a. Conscious procedures

i. Local anesthesia is described as a loss of sensation in a localized area by an anesthetic agent that blocks the neurotransmission of impulses to the brain. It is the backbone of pain and anxiety management. We also know that it is the needle that serves as a primary source of the fear and anxiety we continuously attempt to manage.[32]

ii. Oral sedation or more appropriately premedication describes a route of administering pharmacosedative agents for the purpose of relaxing an apprehensive individual without producing unconsciousness.[33] Administering drugs orally is universally accepted by the general population. Patient cooperation is necessary but usually not problematic, except with children in some cases. Oral medication has a latent period of 30 minutes, peaking at approximately 1 hour, and may be affected by gastric contents. Duration of action and recovery are prolonged, and an escort is often required. There is no mechanism for titration with oral premedication.

iii. Intramuscular (IM) sedation is a method of administering a drug directly into the circulatory system. Clinical action is more rapid than the oral route, and absorption is more reliable. Disadvantageous factors are the inability to titrate the drug, prolonged duration, incomplete recovery, and the necessity of an injection on a cooperative patient.

iv. Inhalation sedation offers the best advantages with few if any disadvantages. These aspects are described in greater detail in Chapter 3, which outlines the rationale for inhalation sedation using N_2O/O_2.

v. Intravenous (IV) conscious sedation has gained popularity because many disciplines are providing appropriate education to predoctoral students. IV sedation affords many advantages over other methods but also implies greater liability to the practitioner. With IV sedation the onset of action is less than 1 minute, with peak effects appearing within that first minute up to 20 minutes. The duration of action depends on the drug being administered. Recovery is incomplete, and an escort is mandatory. The most advantageous aspect of IV sedation is that titration is possible. A disadvantage is the lack of available educational programs.

b. Unconscious procedures

i. Deep sedation refers to IV sedation in which the level of sedation is increased while the patient is

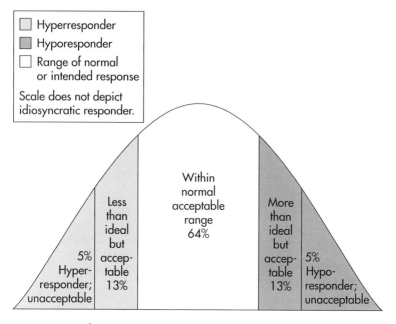

Figure 2-6   Range of individual biovariability.

unconscious. The advantages and disadvantages are primarily the same for IV unconscious sedation as for IV conscious sedation; however, careful monitoring is critical because deeper levels of sedation are easily achieved. This so-called deep sedation is potentially dangerous when general anesthetic agents are used for this purpose.

ii. General anesthesia has been used extensively in the health professions since the discovery of N_2O and ether as anesthetics. Patient cooperation is not a factor for its effectiveness and is often the reason why this modality is selected. Patients who are unmanageable for any reason are candidates for general anesthesia. To perform this technique the practitioner must complete additional educational requirements and assume greater liability.

B. Whichever option is chosen, careful and competent decision-making skills are vital. It is essential to treat each patient as an individual, taking into account the concept of individual biovariability. This concept is based on the premise that no two individuals react the same way in response to a drug or treatment modality. What works for one will not necessarily work for another, nor will one patient respond in the same way on different days.

1. As each drug is initially tested, researchers commonly find a small percentage of hypo- and hyper-responders. Certain people will have no effect from an optimal dose of the drug, while some will incur dramatic effects. A drug is useful when the desired outcome occurs in a large majority of the population without unwanted side effects. Figure 2-6 depicts the range of individual bio-variability.

2. Individual biovariability holds true for nonpharmacologic methods as well. It is wise to keep an open, informed mind while experimenting with pain/anxiety management options. When one modality is insufficient or undesirable, another may prove effective.

C. Select the management option that best suits the situation at hand. As each person responds differently to nonpharmaco-logic and pharmacologic modalities, remember also how variable one's responses are on any given day. Psychologic and physiologic factors must be considered at each meeting with the patient. N_2O/O_2 sedation provides the opportunity to individualize patient treatment with a safe, physiologically nonthreatening, titratable substance.

REFERENCES

1. Thomas CL editor: *Taber's cyclopedic medical dictionary*, Philadelphia, 1997, FA Davis.
2. Consensus Conference: Anesthesia and sedation in the dental office, *J Am Med Assoc* 254:1073-1076, 1985.
3. Stoelting RK: *Pharmacology and physiology in anesthetic practice*, ed 2, Philadelphia,1991, JB Lippincott.
4. Melzack R, Wall P: Pain mechanisms: a new theory, *Science* 150:971-979, 1965.
5. Bell WE: *Orofacial pains: classification, diagnosis, management*, ed 3, St Louis, 1985, Mosby.
6. Hirst M: The changing nature of pain control: clinical aspects of endorphins and enkephalins, *J Canadian Dent Assoc* 51:493-498, 1985.
7. Hargreaves KM, Dubner R: Mechanisms of pain and analgesia. In Dionne RA, Phero JC, editors: *Management of pain and anxiety in dental practice*, New York, 1991, Elsevier Science Publishing.
8. Reisine T, Pasternak G: Opioid analgesics and antagonists. In Hardman JG, Limbird LE, editors: *Goodman and Gillman's: the pharmacologic basis of therapeutics*, ed 9, New York, 1996, McGraw-Hill.
9. Gillman MA: Analgesic (subanesthetic) nitrous oxide interacts with the en-dogenous opioid system: a review of the evidence, *Life Sciences* 39:1209-1221, 1986.
10. Kohr J: Measuring your patient's pain, *RN* 58:39-40, 1995.
11. Gujol MC: A survey of pain assessment and management practices among crit-ical care nurses, *Am J Crit Care* 3:123, 1994.
12. McCafery M, Richey KJ: Techniques of pain assessment, *Nurse Week* 5:16, 1992.

13. Pawlicki RE: Psychological/behavior techniques in managing pain and anxiety in the dental patient. In Dionne RA, Phero JC, editors: *Management of pain and anxiety in dental practice,* New York, 1991, Elsevier Science Publishing.

14. Prins PJ: Anxiety in medical settings. In Ollendick TH, King NJ, Yule W, editors: *International handbook of phobic and anxiety disorders in children and adolescents,* New York, 1994, Plenum Press.

15. Mendola P, O'Shea RM, Zielezny MA: Validity and reliability of the interval scale of anxiety response, *Anesth Prog* 34:202-206, 1987.

16. Parkin SF: The assessment of two dental anxiety rating scales for children, *J Dent Child* 55:269-272, 1988.

17. Elter JR, Strauss RP, Beck JD: Assessing dental anxiety, dental care use and oral status in older adults, *J Am Dent Assoc* 128:591-597, 1997.

18. Weinstein P, Nathan JE: The challenge of fearful and phobic children, *Dent Clin North Am* 32:667-682, 1988.

19. Ketchum C: Freedom from fear, *RDH* 3:14-17, 1995.

20. Alifimoff JK, Miller KW: Mechanism of action of general anesthetic agents. In Rogers M, et al, editors: *Principles and practice of anesthesiology,* St Louis, 1993, Mosby.

21. Snow J: *On the inhalation of the vapor of ether in surgical operations,* London, 1847, John Churchill.

22. Guedel AE: *Inhalation anesthesia,* ed 2, New York, 1951, Macmillan.

23. Gillespie NA: Signs and reflex reactions of stages of anesthesia, *Anesth Anal* 22:275-283, 1943.

24. Stracher K: The role of suggestion in conscious-sedation, *Anesth Prog* 23:59,66, 1976.

25. Ross ID: Fear control with nitrous oxide sedation, *SAAD Digest* 9:69, 1992.

26. Simpson MA et al: *Hypnosis in dentistry: a handbook for clinical use,* Springfield, Ill, 1985, Charles C Thomas Publisher.

27. Malamed SF: *Handbook of local anesthesia,* ed 4, St Louis, 1997, Mosby.

28. Clark MS et al: An evaluation of the clinical analgesia/anesthesia efficacy on acute pain using the high frequency neural modulator in various dental settings, *Oral Surg* 63:501-505, 1987.

29. Christensen GJ: Electronic anesthesia: research and thoughts, *J Calif Dent Assoc* 15:46-48, 1987.

30. Hochman R: Neurotransmitter modulator (TENS) for control of dental operative pain, *J Am Dent Assoc,* 116:208-212, 1988.

31. Malamed SF et al: Electronic dental anesthesia for restorative dentistry, *Anesth Prog* 36:195-198, 1989.

32. Milgrom P et al: Four dimensions of fear of dental injections, *J Am Dent Assoc* 128:756-762, 1997.

33. Malamed SF: *Sedation: a guide to patient management,* ed 3, St Louis, 1995, Mosby.

SUGGESTED READINGS

Heitkemper T, Layne C, Sullivan DM: Brief treatment of children's dental pain and anxiety, *Percept Mot Skills* 76:192-194, 1993.

Kaufman E, Jastak JT: Sedation for outpatient dental procedures, *Compend Dent* 16:462-479, 1995.

Nathan JE: Management of the difficult child: a survey of pediatric dentists' use of restraints, sedation and general anesthesia, *J Dent Child* July/Aug:293-301, 1989.

Slavin HC: What we know about pain, *J Am Dent Assoc* 127:1536-1541, 1996.

3

Comparison of Nitrous Oxide/Oxygen Sedation with Other Sedation Methods

Nitrous oxide/oxygen (N_2O/O_2) sedation has many advantages over other pain and anxiety management options. There are many indications for its use and the disadvantages are few; for these reasons many have labeled it the ideal sedative method. The majority of these advantages deal with the pharmacokinetics of the drug itself. Of course N_2O is not appropriate for every person or every situation. Judge for yourself how the N_2O/O_2 option compares with others.

I. Comparative Analysis of N_2O/O_2 Therapy with Other Methods

A. Analgesic properties (pain control)

1. Chapman, Arrowood, and Beecher[1] state that a mixture of 20% N_2O and 80% O_2 has the same analgesic equipotence as 15 mg of morphine. Pirec, Patterson, and Thapar[2] determined that subacute concentrations of N_2O could reduce cold pressor-induced pain.

2. The level of pain control afforded by N_2O can vary from patient to patient because of individual biovariability; however, the analgesic properties of N_2O are well recognized and its potency is significant.[1] These analgesic properties are useful even with the severe pain associated with myocardial infarction. N_2O may not be sufficient to obtund all pain but its analgesic potential is significant.

3. N_2O/O_2 is also advantageous when other analgesic drugs are contraindicated (i.e., allergy).

4. Fear affects an individual's ability to tolerate pain; painful stimuli can be exaggerated in an anxious patient. A common fear is fear of an injection or a needle (i.e., vaccination), which can intensify an individual's reaction to pain. N_2O has the ability to manage both pain and fear.

B. Anxiolytic properties (sedative effects)
1. A person's mental ability to cope with certain situations can depend on simple things, such as age, stress, fatigue, or illness. Many times patients are anxious about even undergoing diagnostic testing, much less the treatment that may ensue.
2. N_2O/O_2 therapy can significantly assist a patient in handling his/her fear or anxiety by producing sedation or a sense of well-being. Sedation enables the patient to become calm, relaxed, and able to tolerate the situation better or with no difficulty. This relaxed feeling has a positive effect on the patient's pain threshold.
3. In treatment of pediatric patients, N_2O/O_2 has been shown to facilitate positive behavior and lowered anxiety levels on sequential visits.[3] It is a continuing goal of all healthcare professionals to prevent negative early childhood experiences in order to reduce the number of fearful adults. Ultimately, the goal is to provide the patient with enough positive experiences that he/she does not require N_2O/O_2 sedation in the future.

C. Amnestic properties
1. The amnestic property of N_2O/O_2 sedation is another of its positive attributes. Postoperatively, patients often state they cannot recall the severity of their pain or anxiety or its duration.
2. Passage of time tends to become unclear under N_2O/O_2 sedation. A patient may remark how quickly time passed during a time-intensive procedure.

D. Onset of action
1. N_2O/O_2 sedation has a rapid onset of action. Because of the pharmacologic characteristics of N_2O, clinical effects may begin in less than 30 seconds, with peak effects occurring in less than 5 minutes.
2. The only other conscious-sedative modality that closely parallels the rapid onset of clinical action of N_2O/O_2 is IV sedation.

E. Titration
1. Titration is the process of administering a drug incrementally to a specific level or endpoint of sedation. It allows for the exact amount of the drug to be delivered to every patient at every appointment. Titration is very easily accomplished with N_2O/O_2 sedation. In fact N_2O/O_2 accommodates the concept of titration more than any other drug. See Chapter 12.

    2. The only other conscious-sedative technique in which titration is possible is IV sedation, but even then the drug cannot quickly or easily be decreased.

F. Recovery

    1. Inhalation of N_2O/O_2 is the only pharmacologic sedative technique in which there is complete recovery within a minimum 3- to 5-minute period after termination of the drug. Recovery will be discussed further in Chapter 15.

II. Combining N_2O/O_2 Sedation with Other Methods

A. N_2O/O_2 sedation is enhanced with sophrology, the science of the spoken word. Soothing, calm, encouraging words and actions of the operator facilitate the relaxing effects of the drug.

B. Weinstein and Nathan[4] indicate that N_2O used in combination with distraction techniques was more effective than distraction with a placebo gas when working with children. They also suggest that the combination of N_2O/O_2 and hypnosis and imagery were effective with their population.[4]

C. Another combination cited as effective with pediatric patients is the use of audioanalgesia and N_2O/O_2. The addition of music as an adjuvant to N_2O/O_2 sedation was positive for the children studied.[5] Music has been used as a method for calming, relaxing, and distracting individuals in the health-care setting since the era of "white sound" in the late 1950s and early 1960s.[6,7]

D. Quarnstrom[8] was successful in his research when he combined N_2O/O_2 and electronic dental anesthesia (EDA), compared with using each modality alone.

E. Oral premedication may be used safely with N_2O/O_2 sedation.[9] Diazepam and meperidine hydrochloride have been cited as drugs used concomitantly with N_2O.

F. The combination that deserves special attention is that of N_2O/O_2 and local anesthesia. The benefits of local anesthesia are great; N_2O/O_2 should not be used as a substitute for local anesthesia but rather as an adjuvant to it. If N_2O/O_2 is administered solely in a situation that otherwise would require local anesthesia, the patient may blame the N_2O/O_2 unfairly for not eliminating the pain. The patient will be less likely to trust N_2O/O_2 in the future. Local anesthesia and N_2O/O_2 combined offer a superior pain/anxiety management option.

REFERENCES

1. Chapman WP, Arrowood JG, Beecher HK: The analgesic effects of low concentrations of nitrous oxide compared in man with morphine sulphate, *J Clin Invest* 22:871-875, 1943.
2. Pirec V, Patterson TH, Thapar P: Effects of subanesthetic concentrations of nitrous oxide on cold-pressor pain in humans, *Pharm Biochem Behav* 51:323-329, 1995.
3. Veerkamp JS et al: Anxiety reduction with nitrous oxide: a permanent solution? *J Dent Child* 62:44-48, 1995.
4. Weinstein P, Nathan JE: The challenge of fearful and phobic children, *Dent Clin North Am* 32:667-682, 1988.
5. Anderson WD: The effectiveness of audio-nitrous oxide-oxygen psychosedation on dental behavior of a child, *J of Pedodontics* 5:3-21, 1980.
6. Gardner, Licklider: Auditory analgesia in dental operation, *J Am Dent Assoc* 59:1144-1150, 1959.
7. Robson, Davenport: The effects of white sound and music upon superficial pain threshold, *Can J Anaesth* 9:105-108, 1962.
8. Quarnstrom FC: Clinical experience with TENS and TENS combined with nitrous oxide-oxygen, *Anesth Prog* 36:66-69, 1989.
9. Jastak JT, Paravecchio R: An analysis of 1331 sedations using inhalation, intravenous, or other techniques, *J Am Dent Assoc* 91:1242-1249, 1975.

4

History and Evolution of Nitrous Oxide/Oxygen Sedation

In this era of sophisticated medicine and high technology it is easy to forget what early medical scientists went through to advance standard practices such as nitrous oxide/oxygen (N_2O/O_2) sedation. What these scientific pioneers accomplished while experimenting with unknown, potentially dangerous materials and primitive equipment is amazing. They often sacrificed their own health and safety for the sake of scientific advancement. It is because of the tenacity of these early medical explorers that we can provide safe and effective analgesia/anesthesia today.

I. Historical Perspectives

A. Discovery of nitrous oxide and oxygen
1. The discovery of both nitrous oxide (N_2O) and oxygen (O_2) is credited to the English gentleman Joseph Priestley.
2. The actual discovery dates of these gases are somewhat in question because of Priestley's own uncertainty about what he had discovered. The time periods cited in the literature vary from 1771 to 1777.[1] During this time he repeated several experiments that ultimately resulted in the gases we know as nitrous oxide and oxygen.
3. Priestley experimented with nitrous air—a mixture of iron filings, sulfur, and water. The end product was a residual gas with considerably less volume than the original nitrous air. He called this "dephlogisticated nitrous air," which is now known as nitrous oxide.[1]
4. During his experiments with nitrous air, he became aware of another gas, which he termed "good air." He found this air to be "fit for respiration," and he titled this discovery "dephlogisticated air," which is now known as oxygen.[1]

B. Inhalation of N_2O

1. Humphrey Davy, at the age of 21, was interested in the field of medicine. Although N_2O gas was allegedly etiologic to many diseases and deadly conditions, Davy ignored the warnings and, in England in 1798, became the first to inhale pure N_2O.

2. Instead of incurring some dreadful plight, Davy found the experience very pleasurable; he became euphoric and felt like laughing. He continued his experiments, saying they produced the "most voluptuous sensations." Other descriptions of his experiences with N_2O included "ideal existence" and "overwhelming joy."[2] Davy published the results of his experiments in booklet form in 1800.

3. It was when Davy experienced diminished pain from a toothache while using N_2O that he began to believe it could affect pain sensations. This was the first indication of the anesthetic properties of the gas. Davy had no idea of the significance of this experience.

4. For the next 4 decades, experiments with N_2O continued, but not in the medical field. Nineteen-year-old Samuel Colt, posing as a physician, began sporting street corner sideshows featuring N_2O. These shows were touted as a way for young people to enjoy evening entertainment where they could "laugh, sing, speak, or fight."[3] N_2O became the trendy activity at social events and university settings (Figure 4-1). It was the featured demonstration at many lectures.

5. The anesthetic value of N_2O first discovered by Davy was not pursued.

C. Medical world ignores N_2O as potential anesthetic

1. During the early nineteenth century, while reckless use of N_2O continued, the medical community was hungry for pain relief. Surgical procedures often resulted in death of patients for many reasons.

   a. Poor infection control led to secondary infections.

   b. Doctors were unsure of anatomy.

   c. The lack of pain control was problematic.

2. The most commonly performed operations were amputations, tooth extractions, and abscess draining. These surgeries were completed within minutes and often in less than 90 seconds. However, during more lengthy procedures patients would succumb to exhaustion and/or shock.

3. The greatest medical advance at that time was the suture. Wounds could be sewn closed rather than cauterized with a hot iron; extremities remaining from amputations

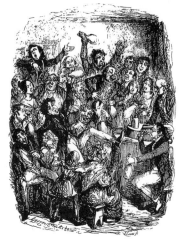

Laughing Gas.

Figure 4-1 "Laughing Gas." (From Scoffern: *Chemistry No Mystery*, 1839. Courtesy of the Harvard Medical Library in the F.A. Countway Library of Medicine, Boston, Mass.)

did not have to be dipped in a boiling solution to cause hemostasis.[3]

4. Prospective patients often committed suicide rather than face an operation without pain control. Pain control measures were time consuming, unpredictable, inconsistent, and at best mildly effective. Several methods were tried.
   a. Brute force to hold a patient down
   b. Preoperative alcohol or opium
   c. Tourniquets, ice, and hypnotism
5. Obviously, prospective surgical patients were often placed in serious dilemmas—choosing between pure torture and unfathomable pain associated with surgery or living with a disease or condition that would more than likely result in a slow, agonizing death.

D. The revelation at Dr. Colton's Grand Exhibition
   1. Dr. Gardner Colton, a New York physician turned professor, hosted the Grand Exhibition in Hartford, Connecticut on December 10, 1844. It was an exhibition to demonstrate the exhilarating effects of inhaling N_2O.[4]
   2. Horace Wells, a dentist, was in attendance. As a participant Wells volunteered to try the gas on stage, believing he would not "make a spectacle of himself." However, that was exactly how Mrs. Wells described his performance.[2]

3. Another participant, a young man named Samuel Cooley, volunteered to inhale the gas in front of the audience. He began to feel the effects of the gas immediately. As he was euphorically jumping around, he hit his leg against a bench causing a deep, bloody laceration. Cooley was unaware of the extent of the injury and professed that he did not feel any pain.

4. Wells was intrigued by the apparent nonresponsiveness of Cooley's pain and asked Colton whether a tooth could be removed under the influence of N_2O. Unaware of any analgesic properties, Colton agreed to bring a supply of gas and meet Wells at his office the next day. There Wells breathed the gas himself and had a colleague, Dr. Riggs, extract one of his teeth. Wells exclaimed "the greatest discovery ever made," and "a new era in tooth pulling." Colton taught Wells how to prepare the N_2O and thought of him as a "visionary enthusiast."[4] Figure 4-2 shows a one-of-a-kind portrait of Wells that appears at the Wadsworth Antheneum in Hartford, Connecticut.

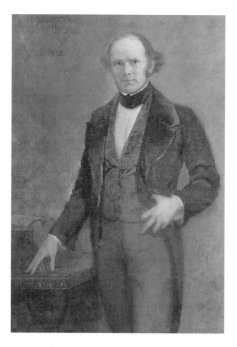

Figure 4-2 Portrait of Dr. Horace Wells, Discoverer of Anesthesia. (Wadsworth Antheneum, Hartford. Gift of Charles Nöel Flagg. Endowed by C.N. Flagg and Company.)

E. The Horace Wells experiment

　　1. Wells used N_2O during extractions on several patients with great success. Anxious to demonstrate this procedure in front of his peers, Wells was allowed to operate in front of several physicians and students in Boston in 1845. As he attempted to remove a tooth, the patient jumped in the chair leading observers to believe he was in pain. Apparently the patient breathed an insufficient amount of gas to prevent him from moving. Some time later the patient indicated he did not experience any pain.[4] Unfortunately for Wells, his experiment was deemed unsuccessful and he was labeled a "charlatan" and a "fake."[5]

　　2. Wells, in his own writings, indicated that he was obsessed with proving the legitimacy of his techniques. He also alluded to being severely depressed over the debacle in Boston.[5]

　　3. For the next several years Wells continued to provide anesthesia for surgeons in the area. Dentists began to give attention to the use of N_2O. In fact, advancing dentistry's reputation hinged on the success of extracting teeth with pain relief.[6]

II. Evolution of Anesthesia

A. Ether anesthesia

　　1. William Morton, a dental student of Wells and later a physician, was present at the famed event presented by Wells in Boston. Recognizing that a more potent anesthetic gas was necessary, he began to work with ether.

　　2. In 1846 Morton performed a surgical demonstration using ether in the Massachusetts General Hospital, later called the "ether dome." (Figure 4-3 shows the ether dome as seen in 1997.) Morton's experiment was similar to Wells's in terms of success; the patient stated that he felt the procedure as it was performed. However, the demonstration was well received by the audience primarily because of Morton's status as a physician rather than a dentist.[7]

　　3. Surgical procedures using ether continued. Other individuals claiming to be its discoverer led Morton to fight for recognition. Morton died in 1848 never having been officially recognized for his accomplishments.

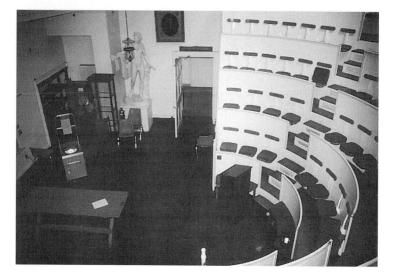

Figure 4-3   The "ether dome" as seen in 1997. (Photo courtesy of Dr. Peter Jacobsohn.)

B. Chloroform anesthesia
1. In 1847 English obstetrician James Simpson was pleased with the anesthetic properties of ether for his patients. However, he did not like the odor or its potential to induce vomiting. He began to use chloroform as an analgesic for labor pains despite others' claims of significant negative consequences.[6]
2. Chloroform continued to be a major anesthetic agent into the 1860s and became standard issue to soldiers who, when injured in battle, could self-administer it.[3]
C. The fight for recognition
1. After his failed performance using N_2O as an anesthetic, Wells's whereabouts and mental status were uncertain for a few years. It was very important to him that he prove his credibility and be recognized for his accomplishments. However, he had become a chloroform addict with unpredictable behavior. Inhaling chloroform contributed to his mental decline and, while in a stupor, Wells threw acid on a prostitute and was imprisoned in New York City in 1848. He asked to retrieve some personal items from his home. A razor and some chloroform accompanied him back to his cell. He wrote his last words to his wife and committed suicide by cutting his femoral artery while under the influence of the drug. At the age of 33 he died

unaware of the credit being given to him while serving his sentence.[5]

2. The Medical Society of Paris, France granted Wells "all the honors of having first discovered and successfully applied the uses of vapors or gases whereby operations could be performed without pain."[4] In Hartford, every physician had signed a document proclaiming Wells as the primary discoverer of anesthesia.[8] In 1864 the American Dental Association (ADA) officially recognized him, and in 1870 the American Medical Association (AMA) proclaimed his honor. Reaffirmation was proclaimed by the AMA on the 100th anniversary (1944) of the original dedication, and in the sesquicentennial year (1994) several dental and anesthesiology societies affirmed once again Wells's significant contributions to the health professions.[8] Also in 1994 he was posthumously awarded the Doctor of Dental Surgery degree from Baltimore College of Dentistry. In addition, a nationwide petition for a commemorative postage stamp (Figure 4-4) was led by Dr. Leonard F. Menszer.[9] Unfortunately, despite thousands of signatures, the stamp has yet to be issued.

D. Resurgence of N_2O

1. The same Dr. Colton who supplied Wells with N_2O in 1844 was responsible for its resurfacing in the early 1860s. Colton insisted that pure N_2O was safe and had an impeccable record of cases to prove it. Between 1864 and 1897 Colton documented 193,000 cases with no fatalities.[6] This began the establishment of its safety record.

2. In 1868 Dr. Edmund Andrews suggested that, when 100% N_2O is used, the blood is not appropriately oxygenated. Andrews added O_2 to the N_2O and claimed one fifth of the volume should be oxygen.[2]

3. Also in 1868 Paul Bert developed equipment to deliver both O_2 and N_2O to a patient.[10] He recommended greater atmospheric pressure when using N_2O/O_2 for human surgeries. However, although his idea was ingenious, it was impractical because of the size and relative immobility of the associated equipment.

E. Twentieth century

1. Dentistry continued to be the primary health profession to use N_2O. However, except for minimal periods between 1913 and 1938, N_2O use was almost nonexistent. Reasons for this inactivity were unreliable equipment, failure to produce satisfactory results, and lack of knowledge of technique.

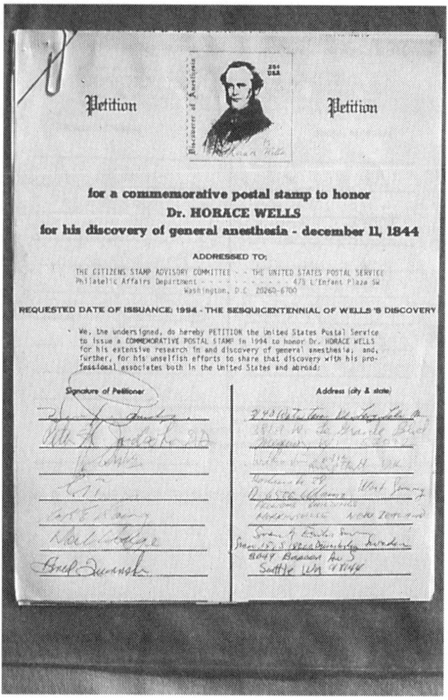
Petition Petition

for a commemorative postal stamp to honor
Dr. HORACE WELLS
for his discovery of general anesthesia - december 11, 1844

ADDRESSED TO:

THE CITIZENS STAMP ADVISORY COMMITTEE - - THE UNITED STATES POSTAL SERVICE
Philatelic Affairs Department - - - - - - - - - - - 475 L'Enfant Plaza SW
Washington, D.C. 20260-6700

REQUESTED DATE OF ISSUANCE: 1994 - THE SESQUICENTENNIAL OF WELLS'S DISCOVERY

We, the undersigned, do hereby PETITION the United States Postal Service to issue a COMMEMORATIVE POSTAL STAMP in 1994 to honor Dr. HORACE WELLS for his extensive research in and discovery of general anesthesia, and, further, for his unselfish efforts to share that discovery with his professional associates both in the United States and abroad:

Signature of Petitioner	Address (city & state)

Figure 4-4 Petition for commemorative stamp, 1994. (Photo courtesy of Dr. Peter Jacobsohn.)

2. Cyclopropane was discovered in 1929 and was subsequently used in the clinical setting as a general anesthetic. It remained the most popular agent for general anesthesia for the next 30 years until its decline because of flammability issues.[7]
3. Medical residencies in the 1930s included N_2O information in their curricula. Anesthesia became a specialty in 1941.[6] Dr. Harry Langa, an early proponent of N_2O/O_2, began postgraduate dental education in 1949.[2]
4. Physicians were not satisfied with the availability and effectiveness of IV agents until sodium thiopental (barbiturate) was deemed acceptable in 1935.[7]
5. Curare was used by anesthesiologists in the 1940s to provide muscle relaxation with light levels of sedation during surgery. When curare was used with N_2O, the incidences of mortality and morbidity were decreased. This combination became the anesthetic of choice for high-risk patients because it did not threaten the cardiovascular system.[7]

6. The century's fourth decade also brought local anesthesia to dentistry, which revolutionized pain control in that setting.[11] Because of the popularity of local anesthesia, it temporarily diminished the use of N_2O. When the role of N_2O was revised to assist with the management of anxiety, its popularity began to rise again.

7. The nonflammable anesthetic agent halothane was introduced in 1956.[7] This introduced a whole new era of anesthetic techniques. It was highly regarded in the medical community because of the minimal side effects associated with its use. This offered a great improvement over other general anesthetics at the time. N_2O was used as an adjuvant drug to enhance the effects of halothane.

8. N_2O remained functional and was commonly used for general anesthesia as a way to provide rapid induction of other more potent agents.

9. Dental schools began teaching the concepts of inhalation sedation in the late 1950s and early 1960s. In 1962 guidelines for teaching pain and anxiety control in dentistry were established by the American Dental Society of Anesthesiology. Today this organization remains at the cutting edge, developing new drugs, techniques, and training for dentists in the area of anesthesia. N_2O continues to be popular in the field of dentistry; approximately 56% of general dentists and 85% of oral and maxillofacial surgeons use it in their clinical practice.[12]

10. Trends followed in other disciplines. Great Britain began using it in emergency medicine and for labor and delivery.[13] Podiatry first cited its use in the literature in 1966.[14] Many other health professions have begun using N_2O/O_2 sedation as a treatment modality for procedures not requiring or inappropriate for general anesthesia.

11. Market predictions show an increase in the consumption of N_2O in the near future.[15] The popularity of N_2O has waxed and waned over the years; however, it has remained in continuous use longer than any other drug. In spite of the advent of other attractive agents, N_2O has never been replaced.

REFERENCES

1. Smith WDA: *Under the influence: a history of nitrous oxide and oxygen anaesthesia,* London, 1982, Macmillan Publishers Ltd.
2. Langa H: *Relative analgesia in dental practice: inhalation analgesia with nitrous oxide,* Philadelphia, 1968, WB Saunders.

3. Fenster JM: How nobody invented anesthesia, *Invention & Technology* Summer: 24-35, 1996.

4. Jacobsohn PH: Dentistry's answer to "the humiliating spectacle": Dr. Wells and his discovery, *J Am Dent Assoc* 125:1576-1581, 1994.

5. Menczer LF, Mittleman M, Wildsmith JA: Horace Wells, *J Am Dent Assoc* 110:773-776, 1985.

6. Chancellor JW: Dr. Wells' impact on dentistry and medicine, *J Am Dent Assoc* 125:1585-1589, 1994.

7. Kennedy SK, Longnecker DE: History and principles of anesthesiology. In Hardman JG, Limbird LE, editors: *Goodman and Gillman's: the pharmacologic basis for therapeutics,* NewYork, 1996, McGraw-Hill.

8. Jacobsohn PH: What others said about Wells, *J Am Dent Assoc* 125:1583-1584, 1994.

9. Jacobsohn PH: Remembering Dr. Menszer, *J Am Dent Assoc* 125:1582, 1994.

10. MacAfee KA: Nitrous oxide. I. Historical perspective and patient selection, *Compend Contin Educ Dent* 10:352-356, 1989.

11. Malamed SF: Local anesthetics: dentistry's most important drugs, *J Am Dent Assoc* 125:1571-1576, 1994.

12. ADA Survey Center: 1994 quarterly survey of dental practice, 3rd quarter.

13. Baskett PJF, Bennett JA: Pain relief in hospital: the more widespread use of nitrous oxide, *Br Med J* 2:509-511, 1971.

14. Arancia L: Nitrous oxide inhalation analgesia in ambulatory foot surgery, *J Am Coll Foot Surg* 5:111, 1966.

15. Frost & Sullivan, Inc: Anesthesia, gas monitoring markets to grow slightly, top $600 million by 2000, *Anesth Prog* 41:64-65, 1994.

5

Multidisciplinary Application of Nitrous Oxide/Oxygen Sedation

Some health disciplines have been using nitrous oxide/oxygen (N_2O/O_2) sedation for mild-to-moderate pain control and anxiety relief for many years. Other healthcare professionals have recently revisited its use, not as a general anesthetic, but as an effective analgesic/sedative for the many ambulatory and outpatient procedures being performed today.

Articles referring to N_2O/O_2 sedation in obstetrics are found in the literature because of long-standing use in Great Britain and the United States.[1] Emergency care personnel, in both the field and the hospital setting, have also been long-term providers of this therapy.[2] Other disciplines have limited literature citations.

Today all health disciplines are providing more patient care services on an outpatient or ambulatory basis. No doubt because of advances in technology, managed care, and the ever-changing insurance industry, these procedures will become even more standard. N_2O/O_2 sedation is a viable treatment modality for these types of procedures regardless of discipline.

I. Emergency Medicine

A. The ideal analgesic for prehospital care in the ambulance
   1. An ideal analgesic agent for prehospital emergency pain control is one that has properties such as quick onset of clinical action, fast recovery, no effect on level of consciousness, no significant side effects, and no masking of other conditions, which would ultimately interfere with the diagnostic evaluation at the hospital.
   2. N_2O possesses many of these characteristics. Several researchers support this notion or indicate that N_2O is close to ideal.[3-5]

B. Historical use of N_2O/O_2 in emergency medicine
    1. The first self-administered, fixed-ratio system used in ambulance service was implemented by Peter Baskett, from England, in 1969. A mixture of 50% N_2O and 50% O_2 was delivered to the patient using an on-demand system. His idea was that a patient in an ambulatory situation should control his/her own sedation by self-administering this fixed-ratio mixture of gases. Baskett concluded his clinical trials (305 patients with significant decrease in pain and no serious complications) with the claim that N_2O/O_2 was safe and effective for use in emergency medicine.[2]
    2. Not long after the initiation of this type of sedation in England, healthcare providers in the United States began using it for emergency medicine. In 1979 Flomenbaum et al[6] was the first to promote its use in United States emergency departments and to document such use in the literature.

C. Current usage and effectiveness statistics
    1. Recently emergency medical services (EMS) have placed priority on early patient stabilization, safe transportation, and effective communication systems (Figure 5-1). Great strides have been made in these areas, making services to the public safer and more effective. Pain control has always been a focus and is gaining greater attention. The issues of masking symptoms or making conditions worse before hospital access are important considerations in the decision to attend to pain with an analgesic agent.

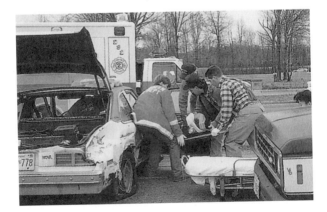

Figure 5-1 Stabilizing the patient at the scene. (From Stoy: *Mosby's first responder textbook,* St. Louis, 1997, Mosby.)

2. EMS personnel continue to use Baskett's fixed-ratio, self-administration technique. This technique is popular because of its portability in the field. Emergency departments in hospital settings may use the fixed-ratio, on-demand equipment or they may use continuous-flow machines like those that have been used in dentistry.

3. Researchers have cited many instances of successful uses of N_2O/O_2 in the prehospital and emergency department settings. Gamis, Knapp, and Glenski[7] completed a study using N_2O/O_2 on pediatric patients requiring laceration repair in the emergency department at Children's Mercy Hospital in Kansas City, Missouri. Thirty-four children participated and were placed in either a treatment group that used a ratio of 30% N_2O and 70% O_2 or a control group using 100% O_2. A clinically significant difference was found in the pain scores between groups of children older than 8 years. Although no statistically significant difference was found with children in the 2 to 7 age group, pain scores decreased when N_2O/O_2 was used.[7]

4. Since then, research projects designed to prove the efficacy and safety of N_2O/O_2 have been sparse, mainly because it has been proved as such for so many years.

D. Indications for use of N_2O/O_2 in emergency medicine[3,4,5,8,9]

1. Many uses have been described in the literature. Examples of procedures in which N_2O/O_2 has been used for musculoskeletal injuries include fractures, strains/sprains, and dislocations.

2. When providing patient care of the skin, N_2O/O_2 may be used when placing and removing sutures; incising abscesses; removing cysts, nevi, or warts; debriding wounds; and dressing burns.

3. Head injuries that are nonneurologic in origin may be successfully treated with N_2O/O_2. Examples are abrasion debridement, removing or draining abscesses or cysts, removing foreign objects from ears, and removing or replacing teeth after trauma.

4. Examples of other procedures include removing or changing drains, catheterization, biopsies, hemorrhoid removal, splinting, extrications, and complicated transfer or movement of patients.

E. Equipment

1. The equipment used in ambulances consists of the gas mixture stored in either a single cylinder or in separate tanks. In some countries the single-cylinder system is

preferred because it is lightweight and easy to operate. A major disadvantage of this 50/50 mixture is the instability of the gases in one cylinder. If the temperature of the mixture is allowed to fall below 5.5° C for even a minimal amount of time, the N_2O will separate and settle to the bottom of the cylinder. A high concentration of O_2 could be dispensed under these conditions, which would mean that pure N_2O would be dispensed as the O_2 is depleted.

2. To date the United States has not approved the single-cylinder system for use. However, this system is popular in countries such as the United Kingdom, Canada, Australia, and New Zealand.

3. A newly marketed product by MDS Matrx Medical Company offers the safety of a double-tank system and the portability of the single-cylinder system. Its major advantage is that it weighs only 11 lbs and can be carried over the shoulder or harnessed to the back. The Nitronox field model is shown in Figure 5-2.

4. In the field setting the patient is required to hold a mask and place it over his/her mouth and nose to inspire the analgesic. If the patient is unable to hold the mask be-

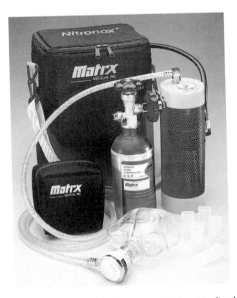

Figure 5-2   Nitronox field model. (Courtesy Matrx Medical Inc., Orchard Park, New York.)

cause of an injury, a mouthpiece can be held tight between the lips and teeth, allowing for inspiration through the mouth. If the patient becomes drowsy, the mouthpiece falls away, discontinuing the administration of the gases.

F. Products

1. The 50/50 gas mixture that is primarily used in the United Kingdom, Canada, and Australia is called *Entonox*. It is manufactured by several companies.
2. Nitronox is available both in the United States and abroad.

II. *Obstetrics/Gynecology*

A. Labor and delivery

1. The literature is saturated with studies reporting manageable, successful labor and deliveries using N_2O/O_2 therapy.
2. A Russian physician began using N_2O/O_2 in 1880 as an analgesic during labor. His experiments led him to the conclusion that it relieved labor pain without harming mother or baby.[10]
3. Swedish literature citations confirm the safety record of N_2O anesthesia. Records show no reproductive problems in nearly 3000 women exposed to N_2O.[11]
4. A 1981 hospital study in Wales evaluated the effectiveness of Entonox delivered through a nasal catheter to women in labor. Both midwives and mothers agreed that Entonox provided labor pain relief.[12] Administration by nasal catheter was comfortable and nonintrusive; however, currently this method of delivery is not recommended because of environmental contamination.
5. A 1994 study in Toronto done by Carstoniu, Levytam, and Norman[13] raised questions about the validity and reliability of previous research on N_2O/O_2 use in labor, citing methodologic flaws as the primary weakness of early research. In the study, relief of pain and oxygen saturation were the foci. Results showed no statistical difference when patients used N_2O/O_2 or compressed air. Patients did recognize the difference in gases, and when offered to continue either, they preferred N_2O/O_2. The oxygen desaturation factor was insignificant, and authors indicated O_2 levels were actually enhanced between contractions.[13]

B. Gynecologic laparoscopy
   1. N_2O has been used for many years as the anesthetic and insufflation agent during gynecologic laparoscopy.
   2. N_2O is advantageous for insufflation because of its non-irritating properties and slow absorption. The American Association of Gynecologic Laparoscopists stated that no adverse incidents occurred in more than 20,000 procedures using N_2O.[14]
   3. The first negative report was in 1979 when Robinson, Thompson, and Wood[15] hypothesized the explosion potential resulting from the reaction of N_2O with methane and hydrogen from the bowel during this procedure. A case was cited in which the patient died resultant to such an explosion.[16]
   4. Although possible, the incidence of such an occurrence is low.[17]
   5. Many other outpatient surgical and nonsurgical procedures in obstetrics/gynecology are being performed in which N_2O/O_2 sedation is the modality of choice.

III. Dermatology

A. Hair transplantation
   1. Hair transplantation is cited as a procedure in which N_2O/O_2 can provide satisfactory analgesia without negatively affecting patient cooperation or producing untoward side effects. Patients in a study by Sadick and Militana[18] responded overwhelmingly (94%) that they preferred N_2O/O_2 over 10 mg Valium and the Dermajet method of lidocaine delivery. Because this surgery requires repeated injections of local anesthetic, the sedative nature of N_2O/O_2 allows for increased patient tolerance.
   2. An N_2O/O_2 advantage noted in hair transplantation is the rapid elimination of the drug vs. others, such as diazepam, which has a longer latent period.[18]
B. Chemical peeling and skin cancer surgeries are also mentioned in the literature as being facilitated by N_2O/O_2 sedation.[18]
C. Liposuction
   1. Liposuction has become a popular procedure. Local anesthetic infiltration has been combined with IM, IV, inhalation sedation, or general anesthesia for this procedure. Professionals state that while many drugs interact with local anesthetics required by this procedure, N_2O/O_2 does not.

2. Dermatologists' experience with N_2O/O_2 is minimal; however, they support its adjunctive properties to local anesthetics.[19] Maloney, Coleman, and Mora[20] concur with others in the dermatology field who support the use of N_2O/O_2. In their study, 46 of 47 patients indicated that they would request N_2O/O_2 for future visits and thought it should be used more in the discipline.

IV. *Podiatry*

A. Ambulatory foot surgeries
1. Ambulatory foot surgery was accomplished in 1966 without incident. It was the first mention in the literature of N_2O/O_2 use in this discipline.[21]
B. Various other podiatric procedures
1. In a 1972 study Mosher and Sorkin[22] provided descriptive evidence of 21 patients requiring varying surgical podiatric procedures while receiving N_2O/O_2 titrated to appropriate levels. No significant side effects were noted; amnesia was reported in 19% of patients. All patients indicated a relaxed sense of well-being. Several advantages of N_2O/O_2 analgesia were listed, one of which was the enhancement of local anesthetic effects.
2. Some of the procedures performed using N_2O/O_2 sedation are digital arthroplasty, nail matricectomy, subungual exostectomy, bunionectomy, excision of digital mass, digital arthrodesis, excision of hallux ossicle, Tailor's bunionectomy, syndactylia, and excision of plantar mass.[22]
C. A more recent (1982) study encouraged specialists to utilize N_2O/O_2 concomitantly with 10 mg of Valium. The authors stated success in more than 150 cases. Their attitude regarding this technique is professed as "a new era in the attainment of near-painless podiatric surgery."[23]

V. *Ophthalmology*

A. Cataract surgery
1. To date, literature citations about the use of N_2O/O_2 sedation in the discipline of ophthalmology are limited. Cataract surgery using N_2O/O_2 sedation is referenced in the *Journal of Ophthalmic Surgery*.[24]
2. N_2O/O_2 is used instead of IM premedication to prepare patients for the necessary local anesthetic injection.

McMahan[24] used N_2O/O_2 therapy on 800 patients for cataract surgery with great success.

B. Implant surgery
   1. Implant surgery performed at the Hawaiian Eye Surgicenter includes N_2O/O_2 as part of the procedure. Professionals there wanted an analgesic/sedative for assistance during the local injection but did not want the prolonged effects of other drugs. They wanted patients to be fully recovered for prompt dismissal.
   2. They expressed satisfaction with the calming, amnestic effects with their 50% N_2O and 50% O_2 technique.[25]

C. Cryosurgery
   1. In cryosurgery, rather than being used for its amnestic effects, N_2O is used to cool metal instruments, which in turn initiates the freezing or tissue necrosis of a lesion.
   2. N_2O is preferred over liquid nitrogen because it is easier to handle.[26]

D. Specialists in the ophthalmology discipline acknowledge interest in the use of N_2O/O_2 sedation in the ambulatory setting.[27]

VI. Neurology

A. Depression
   1. Neurologists have used N_2O/O_2 for patients exhibiting chronic anxiety. Depressed patients found relief from N_2O/O_2 therapy.
   2. In an early study N_2O was found to be more effective than thiopental with electroconvulsive therapy for treatment of depression.[28]

B. Schizophrenia
   1. Traditionally, using N_2O/O_2 with schizophrenic patients has been cautioned because of individual biovariability and the potential for provoking their psychoses.
   2. Gillman[29] found three of four patients became relaxed after N_2O/O_2 use. He documented problems with one patient.

C. Sex research has included N_2O/O_2 therapy as well. Research done by Gillman and Lichtigfeld[30] shows females unable to achieve orgasm became multiorgasmic with therapy that included N_2O/O_2.

D. Migraine headaches
   1. Migraine headaches have been treated with analgesic concentrations of N_2O/O_2. It seems the analgesic and sedative properties of N_2O/O_2 assist with the management of migraine symptoms.

2. In the literature, a 30-minute treatment of N_2O/O_2 titrated specifically to the patient's needs brought total relief within that time period.[31]

E. Miscellaneous procedures

1. Gillman and Lichtigfeld[32] cite that symptoms associated with various other neurologic disorders have been eliminated with the use of N_2O/O_2 sedation. Some examples are Tourette's syndrome, neuroleptic-induced akathisia, and spasmodic torticollis.

2. Gillman and Lichtigfeld[32] refer to these as preliminary investigations that require specific organized study.

VII. *Endoscopy*

A. Gastrointestinal endoscopy

1. One of the most recent N_2O/O_2 research studies done among health professionals is in gastrointestinal endoscopy.

2. Diehl et al[33] presented N_2O/O_2 research results at the American Society of Gastrointestinal Endoscopy (ASGE) 1996 annual session. They indicated success with N_2O/O_2 in the outpatient setting at significantly less cost. In addition, patients generally accepted the procedure and clinicians felt that administering N_2O/O_2 was not problematic and appreciated patient tolerance. The study also looked at differences between using N_2O/O_2 or IV-infused barbiturates. No statistically significant differences were found.[33]

B. These initial results have been met with enthusiasm by a number of specialists in the field of endoscopy. This discipline may be on the verge of opening a new vista in the endoscopy arena.

VIII. *Addiction Withdrawal*

A. Pentazocine (Talwin)

1. N_2O has been investigated as a potential therapeutic drug for addiction withdrawal of certain substances. Kripke and Hechtman[34] were the first to mention this innovation in 1972 when treating pentazocine addiction. Pentazocine is a narcotico-analog analgesic. It is contraindicated for treating patients using narcotics.[34]

2. Pentazocine was used in significant amounts to obviate the continual severe pain of an esophageal (potash) in-

jury plaguing a 14-year-old girl. The patient became addicted to the drug, and clinicians used N_2O/O_2 to wean her from it. Advantages of this therapy were the freedom from pain and the ease of delivery at her home.

B. Alcohol
   1. Lichtigfeld and Gillman[35] found N_2O/O_2 to be effective for alcohol withdrawal in more than 5000 cases in South Africa.
   2. A single 20-minute application of analgesic N_2O/O_2 to a patient during admittance to a treatment center will relieve initial withdrawal symptoms without causing significant sedation, which allows for other social detoxification therapies to be initiated immediately.[35] Other discoveries made using N_2O/O_2 included reduced hospital stays and decreased doses of other medications with no addictive propensity to N_2O.[32]

C. N_2O/O_2 sedation has also been experimented with in treating nicotine and marijuana addiction.[32]

IX. Radiology

A. Painful procedures
   1. Analgesic/anxiolytic N_2O/O_2 has proved beneficial in the discipline of radiology. Pharmacosedation has most commonly been used for many painful radiologic procedures.
   2. In a study[36] of radiologic procedures, 50 of 53 patients reported that N_2O/O_2 sedation improved their procedures. Some of the procedures that use N_2O/O_2 sedation are aortoperipheral arteriography, percutaneous biopsies, visceral arteriography, percutaneous cholangiography, biliary catheter placement, biliary stone retrieval, bilateral ureterastent placement, hepatic artery catheter placement, liver abscess drainage, and bilateral temporomandibular joint arthroscopy.[36] Patients using N_2O/O_2 sedation are far more cooperative when asked to remain still than patients using IV sedation.

B. Magnetic resonance imaging (MRI)
   1. The MRI procedure is often complicated or even contraindicated for patients who are claustrophobic. The procedure requires the patient to be confined to a small space and remain very still for an extended period of time.
   2. Often patients require some type of sedation for anxiety management so that accuracy of the procedure is assured. N_2O/O_2 sedation would be a viable option for this

procedure. However, it may be necessary to explore ways to improve the accessibility of the delivery equipment within the spatial confines of the MRI equipment.

X. *Dentistry*

A. Pain and anxiety
   1. Although local anesthetics revolutionized pain control in dentistry, administering the anesthetic with a needle is still difficult for some patients to take.
   2. Pain and fear are prohibiting factors for seeking dental treatment; more than 40% of the population avoids the dental office for these reasons.[37] N_2O/O_2 sedation offers a way to overcome these barriers.
B. Widespread use in the discipline
   1. Dentistry has been and continues to be a significant supporter and proprietor of N_2O/O_2 sedation. It has been used for several procedures and by virtually all specialties within the discipline.
   2. The dental profession uses N_2O/O_2 sedation for procedures in the areas of periodontics, prosthodontics, orthodontics, dental hygiene, restorative dentistry, oral and maxillofacial surgery, endodontics, and especially pedodontics.[38]

XI. *Pediatrics*

A. Painful and anxiety-producing situations
   1. Pediatric patients present special concerns for healthcare professionals. The more positive healthcare experiences children have, the more likely that they will behave positively during future visits. Also, repeated positive childhood experiences create positive adult attitudes and behaviors.
   2. In spite of a trusting, caring, and kind relationship between a healthcare worker and a child, some procedures hurt. No matter how we prepare a child psychologically for pain, the actual stick with the needle is what they remember. In dentistry, N_2O/O_2 sedation of children has been successful for many years. It is estimated that 88% of pediatric dentists use this method of sedation in their practices.[39]

3. Over a 9-year period Griffin, Campbell, and Jones[40] researched the effect of N_2O/O_2 sedation on more than 3000 children and teenagers in minor surgical procedures. The procedures included laceration/fracture repair, nevi excision, wart removal, abscess incision, and removal of items such as slivers, needles, nails, and fishhooks. Ninety-nine percent of the patients indicated that they would chooese to hav N_2O/O_2 sedation at a future visit. The researchers concluded that N_2O/O_2 has been proved safer than the too-common "cocktail."[40]

B. Amnestic and hypnosuggestive properties

1. These properties are advantageous when treating children. The short attention span of a child often requires additional patient management and time when completing a procedure. The relaxed patient and altered perception of time offered by N_2O/O_2 sedation greatly assists the practitioner.

2. Children are much more hypnosuggestive by nature than adults. A calm, slow, soothing voice facilitates the action of N_2O/O_2 immensely.

XII. *Acute Myocardial Infarction*

A. Reduced pain and anxiety

1. Analgesic levels of N_2O/O_2 have been successfully implemented to relieve acute pain during myocardial infarction (MI). The pathophysiologic process of an MI results in extreme pain and tremendous anxiety. N_2O/O_2 sedation is a perfect antidote.

2. Several studies, conducted from 1962 to 1965 in the former Soviet Republic, proved the effectiveness of N_2O/O_2 with MI.[41,42] Its use in the United States at that time is documented in the literature as well.[9,43] Results of research by Thompson and Lown[44] indicate some relief of pain in 74% of patients. Patients with mild pain were more likely to get significant relief than those experiencing moderate-to-agonizing pain. In those cases, narcotics provided adjuvant analgesic therapy.[44]

B. Supplemental oxygen

1. N_2O/O_2 proved beneficial for those patients being treated in an ambulatory setting for coronary artery disease by decreasing the myocardial O_2 demand.[4]

2. While the O_2 is critical to the myocardium, the N_2O works as the analgesic/sedative for the patient.[4,9,44]

XIII. *Terminally Ill Patients*

A. Cancer or terminal illness
    1. Patients with cancer or in terminal stages of illness often have unbearable pain.[45]
    2. In such cases the issue of adequate pain control is a primary focus of the patient's family and significant others. They want their loved one to be comfortable in his/her final stages of life or when suffering a debilitating illness.

B. Quality of life
    1. Fosburg and Crone[46] report that some patients continue IV-infused narcotics in conjunction with N_2O/O_2 treatment, while others prefer N_2O/O_2 alone.
    2. A patient may be treated at home with N_2O/O_2 therapy and can often control his/her own therapy. In many instances of terminal illness, the N_2O/O_2 therapy improved patients' moods and appetites, and patients communicated more.

C. Hemodynamics
    1. Long-term N_2O/O_2 therapy has been associated with increased white blood cell counts and interference with megaloblastic activity.[47]
    2. The hemodynamic issues surrounding continuous, long-term use of N_2O/O_2 are obviously not as important as relief of pain and anxiety for these patients in final stages of life.
    3. Again, patient comfort is a top priority; restful, relaxed, pain-free last days are intensely sought by all terminally ill patients.

REFERENCES

1. Minnett RJ: Self-administered anaesthesia in childbirth, *Br Med J* 1:501-502, 1934.
2. Baskett PJ, Withnell A: Use of Entonox on the ambulance service, *Br Med J* 2:41-43, 1970.
3. Stewart RD: *Nitrous oxide sedation/analgesia in emergency medicine, Ann Emerg Med* 14:139-148, 1985.
4. Amey BD, Ballinger JA, Harrison EE: Prehospital administration of nitrous oxide for control of pain, *Ann Emerg Med* 10:247-251, 1981.
5. Pons PT: Nitrous oxide analgesia, *Emerg Med Clin North Am* 6:777-782, 1988.
6. Flomenbaum N et al: Self-administered nitrous oxide: an adjunct analgesic, *J Am Col Emerg Phys* 8:95-97, 1979.

7. Gamis AS, Knapp JF, Glenski JA: Nitrous oxide analgesia in a pediatric emergency department, *Ann Emerg Med* 18:177-181, 1989.

8. Pinell MC, Linscott MS: Nitrous oxide in the emergency department, *Am J Emerg Med* 5:395-399, 1987.

9. Hayes, GB: Relief of cardiac chest pain in the field, *Emerg Care Q* 3:49-55, 1987.

10. Marx GF, Katsnelson T: The introduction of nitrous oxide analgesia into obstetrics, *Obstet Gynecol* 80:715-718, 1992.

11. Santos AC, Pedersen H: Current controversies in obstetric anesthesia, *Anesth Anal* 78:753-760, 1994.

12. Arthurs GJ, Rosen M: Acceptability of continuous nasal nitrous oxide during labour: a field trial in six maternity hospitals, *Anaesthesia* 36:384-388, 1981.

13. Carstoniu J, Levytam S, Norman P: Nitrous oxide in early labor: safety and analgesic efficacy assessed by a double-blind, placebo-controlled study, *Anesthesiology* 80:30-35, 1994.

14. Ohlgisser M, Sorokin Y, and Heifetz M: Gynecologic laparoscopy, *Obstet Gynecol Surv* 40:385-396, 1985.

15. Robinson JS, Thompson JM, Wood AW: Laparoscopy explosion hazards with nitrous oxide, *Br Med J* 3:764, 1975.

16. El-Kady AA, ABD-El-Razek M: Intraperitoneal explosion during female sterilization by laparoscopic electrocoagulation, *Int J Gynaecol Obstet* 14:487-488, 1976.

17. Neuman GG et al: Laparoscopy explosion hazards with nitrous oxide, *Anesthesiology* 78:875-879, 1993.

18. Sadick NS, Militana CJ: Use of nitrous oxide in hair transplantation surgery, *J Dermatol Surg Oncol* 20:186-190, 1994.

19. Klein JA: Anesthesia for liposuction in dermatologic surgery, *J Dermatol Surg Oncol* 14:1124-1132, 1988.

20. Maloney JM, Coleman WP, and Mora R: Analgesia induced by nitrous oxide and oxygen as an adjunct to local anesthesia in dermatologic surgery, *J Dermatol Surg Oncol* 6:939-943, 1980.

21. Arancia L: Nitrous oxide inhalation analgesia in ambulatory foot surgery, *J Am Coll Foot Surg* 5:111, 1966.

22. Mosher MR, Sorkin BS: Nitrous oxide/oxygen analgesia in podiatric surgery, *J Am Podiatry Assoc* 62:142-145, 1972.

23. Harris WC, Alpert WJ, Gill JJ: Nitrous oxide and valium use in podiatric surgery for production of conscious-sedation, *J Am Podiatry Assoc* 72:505-509, 1982.

24. McMahan LB: Nitrous oxide analgesia for cataract surgery, *Ophthalmic Surg* 13:307-308, 1982.

25. Corboy JM: Nitrous oxide analgesia for outpatient surgery, *Am Intra-Ocular Implant Soc J* 10:232-234, 1984.

26. Sullivan JH: Cryosurgery in ophthalmic practice, *Ophthalmic Surg* 10:37-41, 1979.

27. Thompson V: Personal communication, September 1997.

28. Brill NW et al: Relative effectiveness of various forms of electroconvulsive therapy, *Arch Neurol Psychiatry* 81:109-117, 1959.

29. Gillman MA: Analgesic nitrous oxide as a therapeutic and investigative tool in neurological conditions. In Sinha KK, editor: *Progress in clinical neurosciences,* vol 2, Ranchi, 1985, Neurological Society of India.

30. Gillman MA, Lichtigfeld FJ: The effects of nitrous oxide and naloxone on orgasm in human females: a preliminary report, *J Sex Res* 19:49-57, 1986.

31. Stanley A: Migraine treated by inhalation sedation using nitrous oxide and oxygen, *Brit Dent J* 149:54, 1980.

32. Gillman MA, Lichtigfeld FJ: Analgesic nitrous oxide in neuropsychiatry: past, present and future, *Intern J Neurosci* 49:75-81, 1989.
33. Diehl DL et al: Nitrous oxide (N₂O) vs intravenous sedation in upper gastrointestinal endoscopy (EGD): a prospective andomized controlled trial, *Gastrointest Endosc* 43:310, 1996.
34. Kripke BJ, Hechtman HB: Nitrous oxide for pentazocine addiction and for intractable pain: report of case, *Anesth Analg* 51:520-527, 1972.
35. Lichtigfeld FJ, Gillman MA: The treatment of alcoholic withdrawal states with oxygen and nitrous oxide, *S Afr Med J* 61:349-351, 1982.
36. Katzen BT, Edwards KC: Nitrous-oxide analgesia for interventional radiologic procedures, *Am J Roentgenol* 140:145-148, 1983.
37. Overcoming dental fear: strategies for its prevention and management, *J Am Dent Assoc* 107:18-27, 1983.
38. Malamed SF: *Sedation: A guide to patient management,* ed 3, St Louis, 1995, Mosby.
39. Davis MJ: Conscious sedation practices in pediatric dentistry: a survey of members of the American Board of Pediatric Dentistry College of Diplomates, *Pediatr Dent* 10:328-329, 1988.
40. Griffin GC, Campbell VD, Jones R: Nitrous oxide-oxygen sedation for minor surgery, *J Am Med Assoc* 245:2411-2413, 1981.
41. Iosava KV: Analgesic anesthesia with nitrous oxide in pain syndrome caused by coronary insufficiency (clinico-biochemical studies), *Kardiologiia* 5:54-58, 1965.
42. Pekker IL: Nitrous oxide anesthesia with pipolphan pre-medication in myocardial infarct at a first aid station, *Sov Med* 28:103-107, 1965.
43. Keer F et al: Nitrous oxide analgesia in myocardial infarction, *Lancet* 1:63-66, 1972.
44. Thompson PL, Lown B: Nitrous oxide as an analgesic in acute myocardial infarction, *J Am Med Assoc* 235:924-927, 1976.
45. Foley KM: The treatment of pain in the patient with cancer, *CA Cancer J Clin* 36:194-215, 1986.
46. Fosburg MT, Crone RK: Nitrous oxide analgesia for refractory pain in the terminally ill, *J Am Med Assoc* 250:511-513, 1983.
47. Brodsky JB: Toxicity of nitrous oxide. In Eger EI II, editor: *Nitrous oxide, N₂O,* New York, 1985, Elsevier Science Publishing.

SUGGESTED READINGS

Cruickshank JC, Sykes SH: Office sedation, *Adv Dermatol* 7:291-313, 1992.
Edwards FJ: The art of sedation in the emergency department, *J Am Acad Phys Assist* 7:128-133, 1994.
Henderson JM et al: Administration of nitrous oxide to pediatric patients provides analgesia for venous cannulation, *Anesthesiology* 72:269-271, 1990.
Hovorka J, Korttila K: Nitrous oxide does not increase nausea and vomiting following gynaecological laparoscopy, *Can J Anaesth* 36:145-148, 1989.
Miller K: Analgesia: issues and options, *Emergency* 21:16, 18-21, 1989.
Thal ER et al: Self-administered analgesia with nitrous oxide: adjunctive aid for emergency medical care systems, *J Am Med Assoc* 242:2418-2419, 1979.
Toulson S: More than a lot of hot air, *Nursing* 4:23-26, 1990.
Tunstall ME: Implications of pre-mixed gases and apparatus for their administration, *Br J Anaesth* 40:675-682, 1968.
Wertz EM: Pediatric conscious sedation, *Emergency* 25:19-23, 1994.

6

Economic Benefits Associated with Nitrous Oxide/Oxygen Administration

When the subject of economics enters the realm of patient care, many practitioners begin to feel uneasy. Although financial expectations may not be the centerpiece of a decision to pursue a health career, it often is a significant factor. Being financially successful is not unethical in and of itself, although there are those in the medical profession who have abused the system for financial gain. However, there is nothing wrong with caring about people and enjoying the benefits of success. As health professionals we should feel good about the services we provide and be profitable enough to continue to practice them.

I. Economic Reflection

A. The "Golden Age of Medicine and Dentistry," a period of post-World War II prosperity that lasted into the early 1960s, was a time of high demand for services and a shortage of clinicians. This situation assured professionals that their practices would be profitable. Because patients were waiting at the door, schedules became tight and profits became palpable. Unfortunately, time and compassion for the patient were not as important for many as they should have been.

B. As the supply of practitioners began to increase in the early 1970s, the demand for healthcare professionals decreased, as did the patient-to-practitioner ratio.

C. Renewed interest in the relationship between clinician and patient has demanded greater sensitivity to patient problems, payment plans, and scheduling demands and an overall awareness of patient needs.

II. Realistic Economics

A. Today's patients have a greater choice in the overall environment of treatment. If they are not treated considerately in one office, they can more easily than ever find an office that makes a greater effort toward meeting their individual needs. This is the basic economic principle of supply and demand at work. Caring, compassionate, competent practitioners are doing very well and have not had economic setbacks because of "too much competition." Indeed, choice has led to patient sophistication in consumerism.

B. Regardless of the socioeconomic strata or educational profile of a patient, he/she as a human being can easily, quickly, and accurately recognize the sincerity of a clinician. Based on experiences, patients use their intuition to determine whether or not they will continue with a certain doctor and whether or not they will refer that doctor to others. Patients do not necessarily have the ability to evaluate a clinician's technical or decision-making skills; therefore their evaluations are based on the clinicians' personal interactions with them.

C. With the advent of managed care, HMO and PPO programs, and changing insurance issues, our knowledge and understanding of economics becomes critical to survival. Clearly, ambulatory services have and will continue to increase because of the regulations placed on time, payments, extent of treatment, etc. Many practitioners feel that these issues have become so intrusive that patient care has suffered.

D. There is no doubt that medicine is changing. We are being challenged to find new avenues for providing patient care with renewed compassion. We may have to advocate our services in a different manner. We may have to rethink our commitment to the profession and to the patient. We may have to become innovative in treatment planning.

E. Patients are always grateful for honest and sincere efforts. In time they will demand the return of lost services and individual decision making. They will stand behind those professionals that they trust. Our practices are truly patient driven.

III. *Dollars and Sense*

A. Do you consider your patients' comfort levels valuable? Are *you* less stressed because you have relaxed, cooperative patients? If so, how much money is that worth? While these and other rhetorical questions may be intangible, a more concrete question is, "How much money can you truly save or earn using nitrous oxide/oxygen (N_2O/O_2) sedation in your practice?" Box 6-1 shows the income potential of using N_2O/O_2 sedation.

BOX 6-1
Income Potential Using N_2O/O_2 Sedation

N_2O at \$30 per visit

Weekly:	Twice per week	=	\$60
	Once per day	=	\$150
	Twice per day	=	\$300
Monthly:	Twice per week monthly	=	\$240
	Once per day monthly	=	\$600
	Twice per day monthly	=	\$1200
Yearly:	Once per day	=	\$7200

Note: Average fee for N_2O (short procedure) is \$50.00.
Figures based on E-cylinders.

B. The actual cost savings or money-making potential of using N_2O/O_2 sedation varies with certain factors. Patient numbers will increase, and time efficiency will be enhanced. These factors alone will increase bottom-line figures proportionally.

  1. An initial decision must be made as to what type of N_2O/O_2 system will be the most beneficial and cost effective. Table 6-1 compares the central gas supply system with the portable gas supply system.

     a. Obviously, if you intend to make N_2O/O_2 sedation common practice in your setting, you may consider a central supply system.

        i. This system allows for multiple flowmeters to be placed in several rooms. Piping and connecting is done within the structure; therefore moving machines and hoses from room to room is not necessary.

        ii. This type of system allows for larger quantities of gas to be stored in a remote location. Larger cylinders, capable of storing more gas, are much less expensive than smaller ones. (See Chapter 7 for more information regarding cylinder sizes.)

     b. Individual, portable units are also available. Practitioners may choose this option as personal preference, especially when only occasionally using N_2O/O_2 and when confines of the physical structure will not allow for a central system.

        i. The entire portable system is on a rolling stand and may be moved from room to room.

TABLE 6-1
Central Gas Supply System vs. Portable Gas Supply System

	Portable System		Central System
Cylinders used:	Small E tanks		Large G (N_2) or H (O₂) tanks
Cylinder volume:	9 E tanks (N_2O)	IN	1 G tank (N_2O)
	10 E tanks (O₂)	IN	I H tank (O₂)
Approximate cost	$12 ($N_2O$)		$48.00 ($N_2O$)
to have filled:	$6 (O₂)		$11.00 (O₂)

If the clinic uses 10 G (N_2O) cylinders and 20 H (O₂) cylinders in 1 year, the savings from using large cylinders would be:

	N_2O		O₂
E tanks:	(9 × $12 × 10)	+	(10 × $6 × 20)=$2,280
G and H tanks:	($48 × 10)	+	($11 × 20)=$700
			Savings=$1,580 per year

Note: Comparison made for U.S. Coast Guard clinic with 10 operatories.

      ii. Gas cylinders for this type of system are smaller, store less gas, and are more expensive than gas cylinders for central systems.

    c. In either situation the initial cost of the N_2O/O₂ equipment should not be a prohibiting factor for its use. This investment will be quickly recovered.

  2. The cost of N_2O and O₂ gases varies considerably in terms of size/quantity of cylinders ordered and distance from a distribution center. Depending on location, costs increase proportionally to the levels of individuals involved with distributorship. Gas costs will most likely be higher the further the distance from a distributor (Figure 6-1).

  3. Patient charges for N_2O/O₂ sedation vary dramatically. They can range from $15 per visit to $80 per visit. Some professionals do not charge the patient for N_2O/O₂ sedation but rather provide it complimentary to the patient. Insurance companies vary as to their payment policies for this service. It is wise to investigate what is considered to be a usual and customary fee according to your most common insurance carriers and local practitioners.

C. Although dollar figures vary between individual situations, N_2O/O₂ sedation will be profitable for your business. Do not discount those figures relating to your profit in goodwill by acknowledging and diminishing your patient's anxiety. Profit is also made by patient referrals. In economic jargon, this is a win-win situation. It just makes sense.

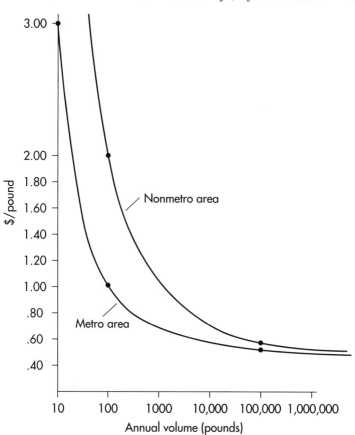

Figure 6-1   Medical nitrous oxide pricing, Metropolitan areas vs. non-metropolitan areas. (Courtesy Nellcor Puritan Bennett, Inc.)

7

Manufacture and Distribution of Nitrous Oxide/Oxygen

XOX

I. Manufacturing

A. Process and storage

1. The manufacturing process of nitrous oxide (N_2O) is relatively simple. The raw ingredient, ammonium nitrate (NH_4NO_3), is supplied as a clear liquid or as solid, pellet-sized particles. This material is used for fertilizer and as a primary ingredient of explosives. Unfortunately, it was involved in the catastrophic bombing of the Alfred Murrah Federal Building in Oklahoma City in April, 1994.

2. To make N_2O, NH_4NO_3 is heated to approximately $250°C$. At that point the NH_4NO_3 decomposes into N_2O, water (steam), and some contaminants ($NH_4NO_3 \rightarrow N_2O + 2 H_2O$). The gas mixture is cooled to ambient temperature, the steam is condensed, and the majority of the water is removed. The resulting crude N_2O gas mixture is scrubbed to extract the contaminants. The gas is then compressed, dried to remove the remaining water, cooled, and liquefied. The resulting product is nearly pure (99.5% to 99.9%) and is stored as a liquefied, compressed gas at 300 psig and 4°F in insulated and refrigerated storage tanks.[1] Figure 7-1 is a flowchart of the steps involved in manufacturing, repackaging, and distributing N_2O/O_2.

3. The manufactured product is kept refrigerated until it is directly transferred by insulated tanker trucks to hospitals with their own large storage facilities or to other gas repackagers and distributors. Approximately 250 gas repackagers and 3200 distributors are in the United States. The dental profession stores N_2O at an estimated 83,700 locations in the United States. The overall medical marketing

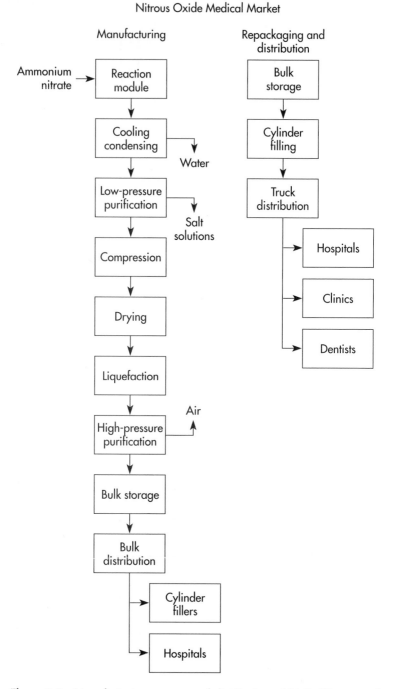

Figure 7-1   Manufacturing process and distribution of N₂O. (Courtesy of Nellcor Puritan Bennett, Inc.)

and distribution system is very effectively and efficiently used in the industry.[1]

B. Users of N_2O

1. Approximately 85% to 90% of the N_2O produced by the six North American manufacturing plants is used in health settings. The majority of this amount (80% to 85%) is used by hospitals to facilitate general anesthesia. The field of dentistry uses up to 10% of the N_2O in ambulatory clinics.[2]

2. The chemical industry uses about 5% of the N_2O manufactured in the production of sodium azide, the explosive agent that inflates an automobile air bag.

3. The food industry uses about 5% to 8% of the N_2O manufactured. N_2O acts as a propellant for dairy products such as whipped cream.[2]

4. N_2O is used to increase engine performance in the racing industry (i.e., cars, motorcycles, boats).[2]

5. It is also used in the silicone chip industry, where it oxidizes chemicals during the manufacture of computer chips. This use requires a 100% pure product.[2]

C. Manufacturers of N_2O

1. The manufacturers of N_2O are: Nellcor Puritan Bennett, Inc., Pleasanton, Calif.; Nitrous Oxide Corporation, Radnor Pa.; and AGA, S.A. DE C.V., Mexico City.

2. Their total output is between 40 and 45 million pounds of N_2O annually.[1]

D. Product expense

1. The entire manufacturing process is relatively inexpensive and provides an excellent product that is affordable for both the healthcare field and industry.

2. The cost analysis of N_2O given in Chapter 6 does not include the costs of filling, storing, maintaining, or delivering the cylinders. These costs vary geographically and depend on the volume requested by the customer, the tank size, and the distance from the manufacturing site to the customer.

II. *Packaging of N_2O*

A. Regulatory agencies

1. The Food and Drug Administration (FDA) regulates the N_2O industry. The FDA has established Good Manufacturing Practices (GMPs) and Quality System Requirements (QSRs) with which companies who produce and

package gases must comply. Compliance with these regulations results in a near 100% pure product, which exceeds U.S. Pharmacopeia specifications.
2. Additionally, the U.S. Department of Transportation (DOT) oversees the packaging and transport of the gas. N_2O is considered a hazardous material and so it falls under the restrictions of the DOT Hazardous Materials Regulations. Cylinders, transportation vehicles, and drivers must meet prescribed regulations. Figure 7-2 shows a driver transporting N_2O/O_2.
B. Storing N_2O and O_2
1. Hospital settings using bulk amounts of N_2O often store the product in large containers. These containers vary in size but range from a 3 3/4-ton to a 14-ton capacity. Obviously, economic cost-savings are of greatest advantage in these situations because the storage, handling, and refilling of cylinders is labor intensive.

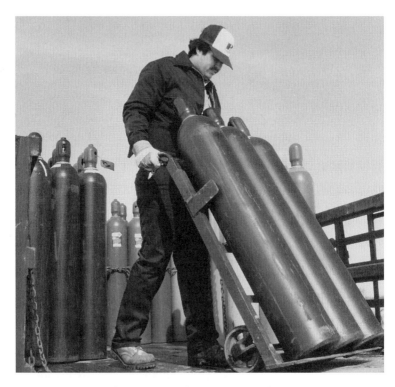

Figure 7-2   Delivering N_2O and O_2.

2. Most often the gas is placed into smaller storage cylinders by a local distributor for delivery.

   a. The metal cylinders are imprinted with critical information such as the origin and age of the cylinder, inspection compliance, and other important data. Figure 7-3 illustrates the top view of typical high-pressure cylinder markings.

   b. The physical integrity of a storage cylinder determines its longevity. It is common to see cylinders 60 to 70 years old in distribution. Aluminum is an alternative cylinder material to alloy steel because of weight factors that affect regulation and cost of delivery. Small, fiberglass-wrapped cylinders offer a lightweight alternative for patients requiring ambulatory oxygen supplementation. These cylinders are the future trend in cylinder construction. Figure 7-4 shows some examples of lightweight and featherweight cylinders.

   c. Cylinders are color coded for easy identification. Color codes are uniform in the United States but may vary internationally (Table 7-1). However, the Compressed Gas Association (CGA) warns that cylinder color may not be a reliable means of gas identification. Instead, the cylinder label provides a more accurate description of the contents.[2]

   d. The size of the cylinder determines the quantity of its contents. However, depending on physical properties of the gas/liquid that is compressed into the cylinder, the amounts will vary. The size of the cylinder has a direct relationship with the economy of its use. Larger cylinders are more cost effective for high-frequency use, and at least twice the amount of O_2 is used per one part of N_2O during inhalation sedation. Figure 7-5 shows examples of several different cylinder sizes.

3. Cylinder storage is important for safety reasons as well as convenience and accessibility.

   a. One of the most important facts to remember regarding compressed gases is that **under no circumstances should grease, oil, or any other lubricating substance come in contact with the gas or gas delivery equipment.** A violent chemical reaction such as a fire or an explosion could occur. When compressed gas pressure is combined with the oxidizing property of N_2O/O_2 and an increased temperature in the reducing valve, the right conditions exist to create a potential explosion.

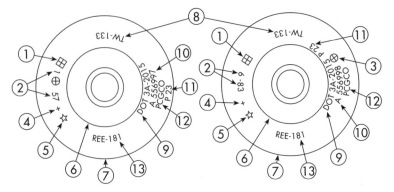

Markings Prior to January 1, 1983   Markings After January 1, 1983

Item	Description
1	Brand identification
2	Manufacturer's test date
3	Manufacturer's registered symbol
4	Cylinder meets 10% overfill specification
5	Cylinder meets 10-year hydrostatic test exemption
6	Collar
7	Cylinder
8	Tare weight
9	D.O.T. specification and service pressure
10	Manufacturer's serial number
11	Inspector's mark
12	Registered owner (PCGCO = Nellcor Puritan Bennett)
13	Rejection elastic expansion limit in cubic centimeters

Figure 7-3 Cylinder shoulder markings detailing various information. (Courtesy of Nellcor Puritan Bennett, Inc.)

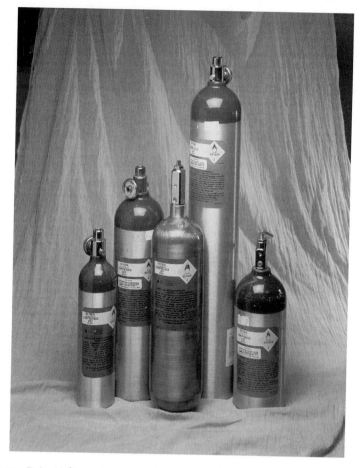

Figure 7-4 Lightweight and featherweight cylinders. (Courtesy of Nellcor Puritan Bennett, Inc.)

TABLE 7-1
Cylinder Color Codes for Various Countries

	N_2O	O_2
Australia	Blue	White
Canada	Blue	White
Germany	Gray	Blue
Sweden	Blue	White
United Kingdom	Blue	White
United States	Blue	Green
Japan	Black	White

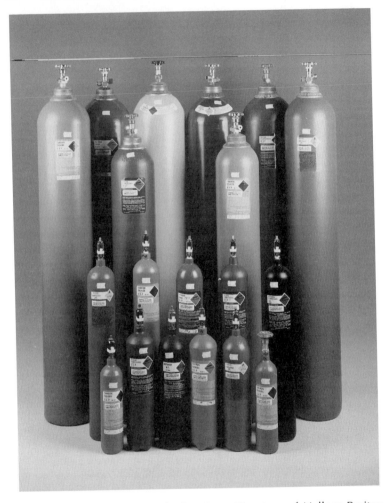

Figure 7-5 Common gas cylinder sizes. (Courtesy of Nellcor Puritan Bennett, Inc.)

b. Larger cylinders associated with a central supply system are stored in an area away from the operatory. Regulations should be followed regarding ventilation and fireproofing of the storage room as well as securing and handling the cylinders.

c. All cylinders should be handled with care and should not be altered. They should only be handled by qualified individuals.

d. Cylinders should be secured in a place that is not readily accessible or visible to others. It is quite possible that persons who abuse N_2O may attempt to locate and access the supply.

3. Requirements for appropriate cylinder storage, installation of equipment, etc. are found in Section 99-C of the National Fire Protection Association (NFPA) code. Additional information from the CGA and the National Welding Supply Association (NWSA) is available. See Appendix A for references.

C. N_2O cylinders
   1. A full N_2O cylinder contains approximately 95% liquid and 5% vapor.
      a. Liquid N_2O in the tank is vaporized by the ambient room air outside the tank as the gas is used.
      b. Because of this heat transfer process, the tank becomes cool to the touch; frost may be seen on the tank surface during prolonged use.
   2. A full cylinder of N_2O will have a pressure-gauge reading of approximately 750 psi at 70° F. If the cylinder is colder as a result of storage conditions or rapid withdrawal, the full cylinder pressure will be less. At a temperature of 50° F, the cylinder pressure will be about 575 psi.
      a. Because the liquid is vaporized as the gas is used, this reading is not proportional to the actual amount of gas available in the cylinder.
      b. Therefore the gauge will show a pressure decrease when the tank contains approximately 20% N_2O. The drop in the dial on the N_2O tank is not proportional to the contents of the tank as with O_2. Figure 7-6 illustrates pressure gauge readings for full N_2O and O_2 cylinders.

D. O_2 cylinders
   1. O_2 is found as a gas in a cylinder. When the O_2 cylinder is full, the amount of pressure is approximately 2000 psi.
   2. The pressure gauge for O_2 will accurately indicate the amount of gas present in the cylinder at all times until the cylinder is exhausted.
      a. The dial will accurately reflect the quantity of gas available in the cylinder for use. If the dial reads 1000 psi, the cylinder is considered half full.
      b. It is important to monitor the amount of O_2 left in the cylinder while it is in use. Because the machine is driven by O_2 flow, if the O_2 tank becomes empty during a procedure, there will be no flow of N_2O and the sedation experience will be interrupted. It is important to have additional O_2 available to prevent this occurrence.

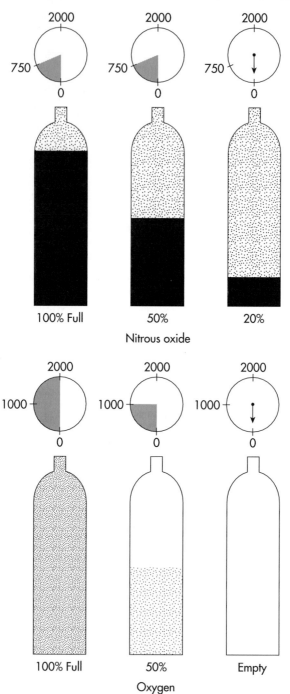

Figure 7-6 Pressure gauge readings for N₂O and O₂ cylinders.

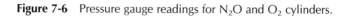

III. *Manufacturers of N_2O/O_2 Sedation Equipment*

A. There are three major companies in the U.S. that manufacture and distribute N_2O/O_2 delivery systems. They are Accutron, Inc., Phoenix, Ariz.; MDS Matrx Medical Inc., Orchard Park, N.Y.; and Porter Instrument Co., Inc., Hatfield, Pa. (See Appendix A for references.)

B. Authors' note: We can personally attest to the genuine concern of each of these companies to manufacture the best and safest products for the mutual benefit of both patient and professional.

IV. *Delivery of N_2O/O_2*

A. History and evolution of N_2O/O_2 delivery equipment
   1. N_2O/O_2 sedation equipment has evolved dramatically since the initial delivery through a bladder bag for Horace Wells.
   2. Sir Fredrick Hewitt in 1887 was the first to incorporate oxygen into a machine that would deliver both gases.[3]
   3. Early machines were designed as intermittent (demand) flow.[3]
   4. A pivotal point in the progression of this technology was the addition of the fail-safe O_2 mechanism in the mid 1970s. This device prevented the delivery of 100% N_2O and assured that no less than 21% (O_2 concentration in ambient air) would ever be delivered to the patient.[3] Today this tolerance is 30%.
   5. Gary Porter, president of Porter Instrument Co. Inc., played an integral role in the evolution of the early analgesia/sedation units. The Porter Instrument Co. is the only company to manufacture the flowmeter glass tubes found in sedation units and hospital anesthesia machines around the world.
   6. Today we enjoy the amenities of audible alarms, digital readouts, tactile-sensitive features, and high-quality performance.

B. Central gas supply system
   1. A central gas supply system is used when a large quantity of gas is supplying several units. Practitioners may prefer this system because of the frequency of N_2O/O_2 use, cost savings, convenience, space saving, etc.
   2. A central-system manifold (Figure 7-7) is a device that connects several large cylinders of gas together and allows

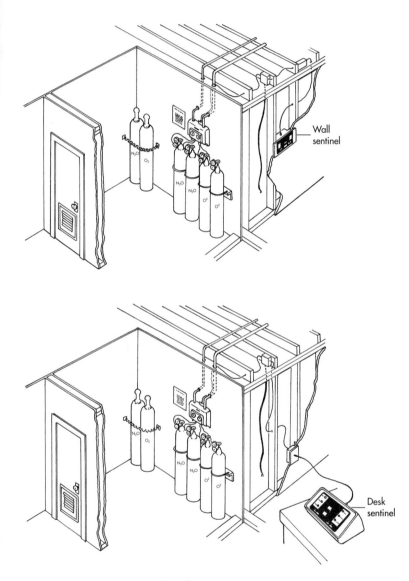

Typical Tank Room Layout

Figure 7-7   Appearance of central manifold.

for the transfer of gas supply from one tank to another when the tank is depleted.

a. A manifold is used to connect a central gas supply to individual operatories and to ensure a constant availability of gas.

b. They can be manually operated or virtually self-automated.

c. Manifold systems are designed to supply gas to as many as 10 units in a given facility. Beyond 10 units, the facility is considered a hospital-care unit and is regulated accordingly.

d. The manifold system is most conveniently and effectively used when it is incorporated as part of the architectural design of the operatory (Figure 7-8).

e. The newest manifolds have several safety features built into the system.

Typical System Layout

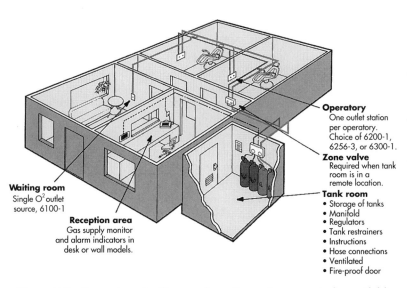

Operatory
One outlet station per operatory. Choice of 6200-1, 6256-3, or 6300-1.

Zone valve
Required when tank room is in a remote location.

Tank room
- Storage of tanks
- Manifold
- Regulators
- Tank restrainers
- Instructions
- Hose connections
- Ventilated
- Fire-proof door

Waiting room
Single O^2 outlet source, 6100-1

Reception area
Gas supply monitor and alarm indicators in desk or wall models.

Figure 7-8 Examples of office configuration using a central manifold system.

      i. Pressure-relief valves will exhaust any gas higher than 75 psi.

     ii. Alarm systems, both visual and audible, will alert a designated person if the pressure of the gas falls below 45 psi or becomes higher than 60 psi. A wall alarm placed in the operatory will alert the practitioner, while a desk alarm will alert an individual at a central location.

3. All gas from the manifold travels through precleaned, degreased copper tubing, and all connections are silver-soldered at 1000° F. The piping system must be pressure tested with nitrogen (N_2) (air) for 24 hours at no less than 150 psi before patient use. Half-inch copper tubing for delivery of O_2 and 3/8-inch tubing for N_2O have become norms. The difference in tubing size prohibits the inadvertent crossing of lines. However, at least one fatality has occurred because of installation errors and subsequent delivery of 100% N_2O instead of O_2. Piping, Industry, Progress, and Education (PIPE) is an organization dedicated to educating users of N_2O/O_2 sedation about the proper installation of the system. See Appendix A for references.

4. For the gas to be dispensed safely there must be a means for reducing the amount of gas pressure from the cylinder. A pressure-reducing valve or regulator is necessary to ensure safe delivery of gas to the patient and through the equipment.

   a. The high pressures of 750 psi in the N_2O tank and 2000 psi in the O_2 tank are reduced to lower pressures of approximately 50 psi.

   b. Regulators are commonly found on the cylinders of central supply delivery systems.

   c. Pressure gauges accompany regulators and have color-coded dials corresponding to the appropriate gas. Gauges display gas pressures within the tank and may not, as in the case of N_2O, indicate the quantity of the gas remaining in the tank.

C. Portable gas delivery system

1. A portable gas delivery system is often used when N_2O/O_2 sedation is not used frequently. The unit houses smaller tanks and may be moved easily from place to place.

2. The yoke stand of the portable manifold is the backbone and supporting structure upon which the equipment rests (Figure 7-9). Stands vary slightly in style; all are easily transportable on wheels.

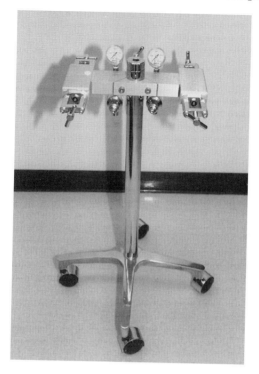

Figure 7-9 Stand and yoke of portable delivery system.

3. The E-yoke is the metal framework adjoining the stand to which the cylinders are attached. There is an attachment configuration for the cylinder to match in order to be correctly attached to the unit. Metal pins, specifically arranged, protrude from the yoke onto which the cylinder is fitted. This precise mechanism is designed to prevent the incorrect cylinder attachment to the yoke and is known as the *pin index safety system* (Figure 7-10).

4. Regulators (Figure 7-11) are found on portable delivery systems for the same reason they are used on central delivery systems. After the gas pressure has been reduced, it is delivered through low-pressure hosing connected to the back of the flowmeter, the boxlike portion of the unit, which contains switches, knobs, etc. (Figure 7-12). These hoses are color coded respectively for the gases and purposely vary in size and threaded end connections to prevent improper gas flow to the machine.

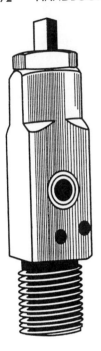

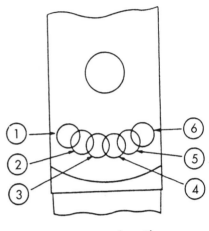

Post type valve with
pin-indexed outlet

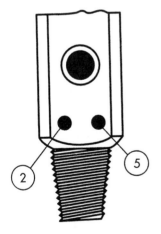

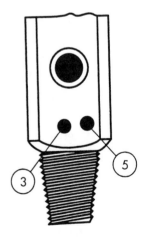

CGA Connection No. 870
Valve yoke connection oxygen

CGA Connection No. 910
Medical cylinder valve
connection nitrous oxide

Figure 7-10   Pin index safety system. (Courtesy of Nellcor Puritan Bennett, Inc.)

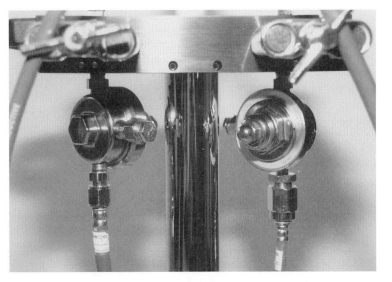

Figure 7-11   Regulators to decrease high pressure from cylinders for patient delivery.

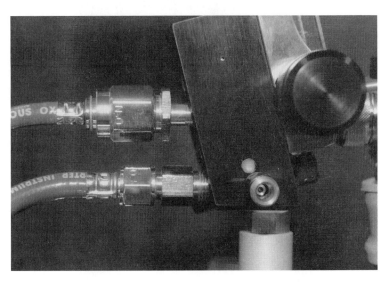

Figure 7-12   Pressure hosing from regulators into flowmeter.

5. At this point, the equipment is the same whether delivering gas from either a central supply or a portable unit.

D. Flowmeter

1. The flowmeter (Figure 7-13) is the unit that sits on top of the yoke assembly and to which the gas hoses are

attached. This highly calibrated device indicates the amount of gas being delivered to the patient.

2. Gas flows into separate sections of the flowmeter and ultimately shows its flow in the gas tubes on the front of the unit. Small balls within the tubes rise and fall according to the amount of gas flowing into the flowmeter. The number corresponding to the middle of the ball indicates the liters of flow per minute of a gas being delivered to the patient.

3. One of the most important safety features of the sedation unit is the flowmeter's fail-safe mechanism. A valve opens to allow N_2O flow only when there is flow of O_2 to the system. Any time the O_2 flow is less than 30%, N_2O stops flowing. This feature prevents the potential

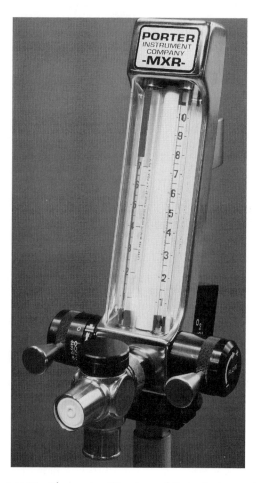

Figure 7-13   Flowmeter. (Courtesy of Porter Instrument Co.)

delivery of 100% N_2O and is standard on every sedation unit made today.

E. Reservoir bag

1. The reservoir bag (Figure 7-14) serves three purposes. Its primary purpose is to provide a source of additional gas should the patient inspire more gas than is being supplied through the hoses. Typically, a reservoir bag holds approximately 3 L of gas. Other sizes are available (e.g., a smaller bag for pediatric patients).

2. Additionally, the reservoir bag provides a mechanism for monitoring the patient's respiration. Watching the expansion and contraction of the bag during sedation assures the operator of the patient's quiet inhalation and exhalation.

3. The reservoir bag also functions in an emergency as a method of providing positive-pressure O_2 to the patient. The bag is gently squeezed to empty its contents into the pulmonary tree; the action is similar to a manual-resuscitator bag. Assisting ventilation in this manner overcomes resistance when accompanied by a full face mask with a tight seal rather than a nasal hood.

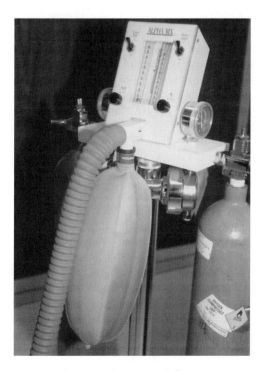

Figure 7-14   Reservoir bag.

    4. Tactile-sensitive materials (i.e., pebble-covered vs. smooth) are available to facilitate easier and more ergonomic manual use.

F. Conduction tubing

    1. Gas is delivered through tubing or hose stemming from the unit and attaching to the breathing apparatus, as shown in Figure 7-15.

    2. Care should be taken to prevent kinking of the hose, thereby preventing gas flow. If this should happen the

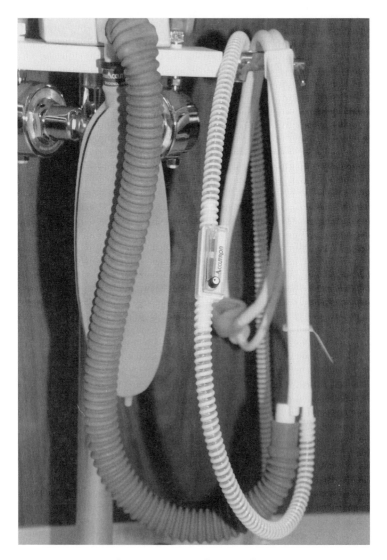

Figure 7-15   Conducting tubing.

patient would most likely alert the operator of breathing difficulty. The reservoir bag will also overfill and balloon because of the constriction of the hose.

3. The concept of anatomic dead space is relative to the length of the conduction tubing. The distance from the gas source to the patient's lungs can increase the anatomic dead space and be lengthened by the conduction tubing. It is important not to add additional hose to facilitate delivery to another area or the other side of the room because of this factor.

4. Units consist of a combination of corrugated and noncorrugated tubing. Tubing diameters vary, with most tubing narrowing near the attachment of the breathing apparatus.

G. Breathing apparatus (nasal hood/face mask)

1. Gas may be delivered to the patient through a nasal hood or a full face mask. Depending on the discipline, one method may be favorable over the other. For example, in dentistry, because of the necessary access to the mouth, a full face mask is not practical.

2. The nasal hood is most commonly used with today's sedation equipment. One of the reasons is that dentistry represents a large sample of the product consumers.

   a. The nasal hood is designed to fit snugly over the patient's nose so that gas does not leak out the sides. There are several sizes available (Figure 7-16).

   b. Accutron, Inc. is the leader in scented nasal hoods. Masks are offered in a variety of scents, including vanilla, peach, strawberry, and bubble gum. Unscented nasal hoods are also available.

   c. The most current models of nasal hoods are disposable and meant for individual use to minimize cross-contamination. Other reusable versions of the hoods are also available but must be sterilized between patients.

   d. Practitioners may choose to sell the nasal hoods to the patient and suggest he/she bring it to the next appointment.

   e. All nasal hoods should have scavenging capabilities. One design provides fresh gas to the hood for the patient through two hoses while two additional hoses evacuate gas being exhaled by the patient. These hoses are connected to a vacuum system that exhausts the gases out of the building. Another system (Figure 7-17) has a scavenging cone on top of the nasal hood to evacuate exhaled gas, which is also attached to a vacuum suction system for external exhausting.

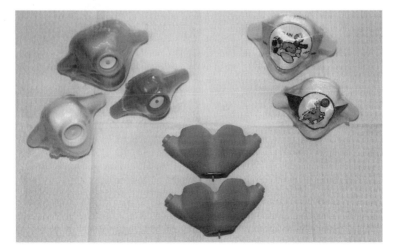

Figure 7-16   Scavenging nasal hoods of various sizes, shapes, and scents.

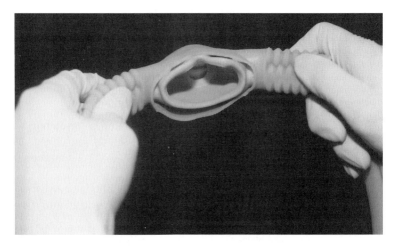

Figure 7-17   Scavenging masks have the capability of providing fresh gas while removing exhaled gas.

  f. It is considered practicing below the standard of care for any healthcare professional not to use a scavenging nasal hood.
3. A full face mask may be used in place of the nasal hood when accessibility to the mouth is not an issue. A piece of elastic usually accompanies the mask and is placed over the patient's head to secure the mask. Because the mask is intended to cover both the mouth and nose, it is much

larger than the nasal hood. Patients may remark that it is claustrophobic by design and may be more anxious about its placement. It is generally used for anesthetic procedures (i.e., general anesthesia) or emergency oxygen delivery.

V. *Infection Control Guidelines*

A. In medicine and dentistry there have been changes in many aspects of healthcare delivery in relation to disease transmission and infection control. Much of what we use is disposable and intended for single patient use. Other supplies and materials have been upgraded to allow for heat/steam sterilization procedures.

　　1. Using disposable nasal hoods is recommended.

　　2. Dispose of conducting tubing, reservoir bags, and nasal hoods when persons with known communicable diseases are being treated.

　　3. Follow manufacturer recommendations regarding sterilization procedures for specific items. Some items can withstand high-temperature sterilization. It is not recommended to place nasal hoods into gluteraldehyde disinfecting solutions. This can cause significant skin irritation.

　　4. Surface disinfection of the equipment is recommended before and after patient treatment. Barriers may be used to cover knobs, dials, throttles, and switches. Bag barriers covering the entire unit may be used as long as they are clear and allow unobstructed visualization of the flowmeter. Evacuation solution, similar to that used to flush and disinfect dental evacuation lines, may be used to flush conducting tubing after use.

B. The various manufacturers will have their own recommended infection-control procedures for the appropriate disinfection and sterilization of products. It is prudent practice to follow these recommendations closely. The manufacturers have researched the parameters of maintaining the integrity of their products; abide by their specifications.

VI. *Variations of Equipment*

A. Design

　　1. Currently, there is a variety of available designs of sedation equipment from which to choose. Manufacturers

determine their own style, color, size, etc. of equipment. However, the design features are similar. Each has common performance features and similar safety features; any variations are in location of the features on the equipment and whether they are manual or automatic.

2. A sedation unit may have separate controls (Figure 7-18), one regulating the flow of N_2O and another controlling O_2 flow. In this case both knobs will be used as the gases are delivered.

3. Another type of unit (Figure 7-19) may be able to mix the gases together and control the total flow being delivered to a patient. This unit is designed to maintain a constant total flow to the patient; gas is increased or decreased using one dial. The percentage of N_2O administered can be adjusted with the dial.

4. MDS Matrx Medical has designed a sedation unit that includes an LED-lighted display panel (Figure 7-20) and an audible alarm system. The mixing unit is controlled with arrow keys for increasing or decreasing gas, and it can maintain a constant liters flow. This machine has many advantages; however, a noted disadvantage is its need for electricity. Battery back-up systems are being researched.

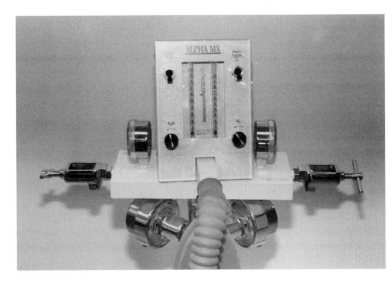

Figure 7-18 Sedation unit with separate gas flow controls. (Courtesy of Accutron, Inc.)

5. Accutron has a newly designed flowmeter, the Ultra flowmeter. In addition to several aesthetically pleasing new features, this machine has the capability of blocking the flow of N_2O with a key lock. This feature maintains the value of the machine as an O_2-delivering mechanism in emergency situations while simultaneously securing the N_2O.

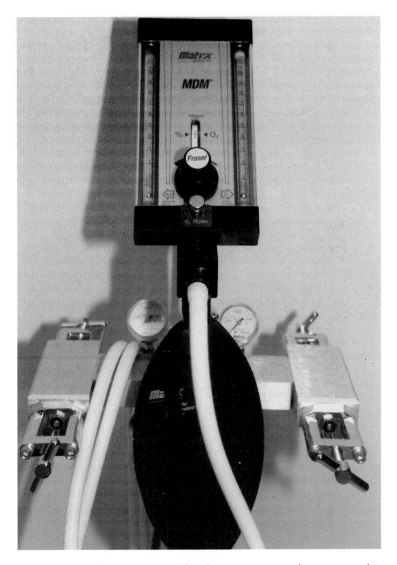

Figure 7-19 Sedation unit capable of mixing gases; only one control is necessary. (Courtesy of MDS Matrx Medical, Inc.)

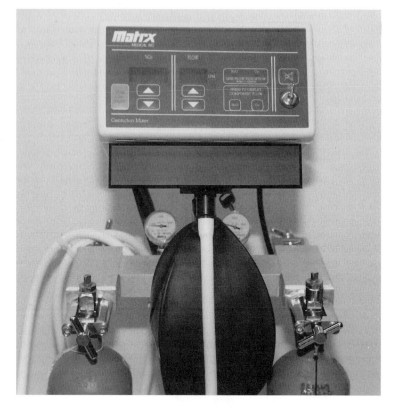

Figure 7-20 Electronic digital display unit. (Courtesy of MDS Matrx Medical, Inc.)

6. An international manufacturer in Japan produces a machine that actually calculates the amount of N_2O and O_2 used for a procedure. In that country the cost of N_2O is quite high ($20 per pound). Consumers are charged for the exact amount (per gram) of N_2O used. The machine displays the amount and subsequent charge to the patient on a receiptlike slip of paper for direct reimbursement to the healthcare facility.

B. Customization
1. Depending on specific consumer needs, manufacturers can customize equipment accordingly.
2. Restrictions may apply regarding the maximum allowable N_2O concentrations able to be administered by some groups, countries, or organizations. Certain military groups restrict concentrations and thus purchase units that have been customized to limit the amount of N_2O able to be delivered.

3. Equipment available for international use varies widely. Depending on the country using the sedation equipment, markings may be customized to accommodate various languages; colored hoses, tubing, etc. may vary depending on the color codes specific to a country.

C. Cost

1. The cost of the necessary sedation equipment should not be prohibitive to providing this service. Expenses should be recovered quickly with patient use and reimbursement of fees.

2. As mentioned earlier, it is necessary to choose the delivery mode according to the frequency of use. A central system is much more cost effective; include it in your building plans if possible. The portable system offers the flexibility of moving it from place to place without the initial expense.

3. Currently, a complete portable system is available for approximately $2500. It is difficult to estimate the cost of a central system because the variables are much greater.

4. Authors' note: We support the products of each of the three major manufacturers in the United States and can ensure the integrity of those companies. See Appendix A for references.

D. Maintenance

1. Manufacturers recommend servicing sedation units periodically. Each company may have specific time frames for maintenance of its units. It is prudent to follow these recommendations to ensure safe delivery to the patient.

2. Servicing a unit includes procedures such as recalibration, pressure testing, internal component checking and replacement, and other factory testing procedures.

3. If at any time the integrity of the equipment is questionable or the unit is not functioning properly, it is important to discontinue its use and alert those who service the equipment. It is critical not to tamper with or attempt to repair any sedation equipment yourself. Leave servicing and inspecting to those properly trained in this area.

VII. *Equipment Safety Features*

A. Several safety features are inherent components of N_2O/O_2 delivery equipment for ambulatory settings. These features provide both patient and professional assurance of the safe delivery of N_2O/O_2 sedation.

1. The most important safety feature of the unit is the O_2 fail-safe mechanism. It ensures that N_2O will not be delivered unless there is O_2 flowing to the machine. Because of this device, the possibility of administering 100% N_2O to a patient has been eliminated. The mechanism's function is based on pressure. O_2 flows into the unit at a pressure that opens a valve to allow the flow of N_2O. If the O_2 pressure drops because of depletion of the supply, the valve closes, thereby preventing the flow of N_2O. This safety feature is standard on every sedation unit manufactured today. Units made before 1976, when this feature was added, should not be used. Using outdated equipment places the operator in legal jeopardy as he/she is practicing below the established standard of care.

2. Currently, the units manufactured in the United States are designed to deliver a minimum of 30% O_2 at all times. It is critical to maintain an O_2 level of at least that in ambient air (21%). The minimum of 30% established by the manufacturers allows for a slight margin of error in calibration. Similarly, the equipment is designed to deliver no more than 70% N_2O at any time. For analgesia and sedation purposes, it is not necessary to administer N_2O concentrations higher than 70%. Caution should be taken whenever concentrations exceed 50%.

3. An index safety system is designed to prevent the inadvertent attachment of the N_2O cylinder to an O_2 portal.

   a. A pin system is used for portable machines in which small cylinders attach to the yoke. Each cylinder of compressed gas has two small holes drilled into the valve stem that correspond to a specific configuration identifying the contents of the cylinder. Two small pins on each portal of the yoke configured exactly with the holes on the cylinder form the attachment mechanism between the cylinder and unit (see Figure 7-10).

   b. On equipment that uses larger tanks, the index system includes thread size and configuration of the valve connection on the tank to the regulator. Again, each gas has a specific configuration to avoid incorrect attachments.

4. With the diameter index safety system the hoses through which the gas travels from the cylinder to the unit are unable to be attached to the wrong stem. The attachment couplings are different in diameter, as are the hoses and stems (Figure 7-21).

5. Near the unit's reservoir bag is an emergency air inlet. This provides an additional source of air for the patient

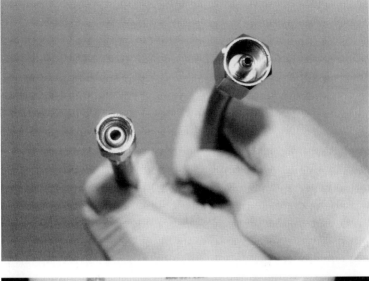

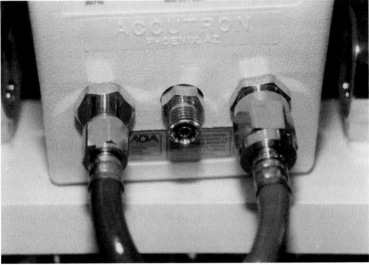

Figure 7-21 Diameter index safety system.

in the circumstance that the reservoir bag is inadequate or the gas flow decreases for some reason.

6. A nonrebreathing valve located near the reservoir bag prohibits exhaled gas from the tubing from entering the reservoir bag. Should this occur, the admixture of gas within the bag would include significant amounts of carbon dioxide (CO_2) that could be rebreathed by the patient.

7. The reservoir bag may serve to assist with patient respirations should an emergency situation arise.

8. There is an auxiliary positive-pressure oxygen hookup on the unit capable of adapting to any quick-connect oxygen supply (Figure 7-22). The sedation unit is indispensable for emergency resuscitation situations.

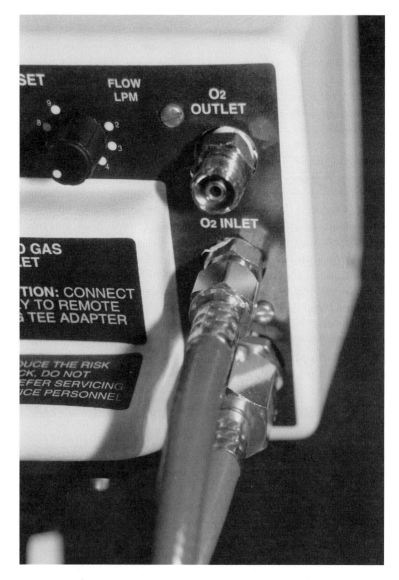

Figure 7-22   Positive-pressure oxygen connection.

9. There are several alarm options, depending on the type of system or unit being used. Alarms can be audible and/or visual to indicate a depleting oxygen supply. Audible alarms are mandatory in Europe and are recommended in the United States.

REFERENCES

1. Fettes WC: Personal communication, August 1996.
2. Compressed Gas Association Code-201, *Nitrous oxide sales and security recommended guidelines,* Compressed Gas Assoc., Arlington, Va, 1995.
3. Compressed Gas Association Code-9, *Standard color marking of compressed gas containers intended for medical use,* Compressed Gas Assoc., Arlington, Va, 1993.
4. Malamed SF: *Sedation: a guide to patient management,* ed 3, St Louis, 1995, Mosby.

8

Patient Assessment

To best serve a patient it is imperative that the healthcare provider obtain pertinent information about the current and previous health history of the patient. This information is acquired during a formal interview with the patient. Undivided attention is necessary to assess the patient's physiologic and psychologic status so that the best pain/anxiety management option may be selected.

I. Health History Information

- A. Upon entering a clinical health facility, the patient is given a form or series of forms to complete. Unfortunately, the most sought after information deals with payment, insurance, agency affiliations, etc.
- B. Questions about health information are often completed by the patient in the reception area, and no further inquiries are made by a practitioner. It is assumed that this information is seen before patient treatment; however, this may not be the case.
- C. Assuming that we are prudent, responsible practitioners, it is desirable to obtain this information through interaction with our patients. Information exchanged through a formal interview process enables professionals to further question responses and make an assessment of patient pain and anxiety. Health histories should be updated at each visit.
- D. It is highly recommended to include a question(s) about pain and anxiety on the health history form itself.[1] This provides patients with a nonthreatening way to communicate anxious feelings that they may be hesitant to divulge verbally. Examples of such questions include: "Is there anything about being here for treatment that bothers you?" "Have you had a previous negative experience in an office/clinic before?" or "Have you previously required special procedures or medication for

nervousness before an appointment?" Scales indicating pain and/or anxiety levels can be included on the health history form as well.

E. Some patients will feel comfortable about communicating their anxious feelings verbally. Others will not admit to uncomfortable feelings but may show outward signs such as sweating, shaking, syncope, etc. In either case, those initial minutes of small talk are valuable for gathering information.

F. A professional can then use the health information obtained from the interview to make an assessment as to the health risk of the patient before performing medical/dental procedures.

II. Assessment of Patient Risk

A. The American Society of Anesthesiologists (ASA) developed a method of classifying patients according to medical risk. This was done to approximate the amount of risk presented by a patient before a surgical procedure. The Physical Classification System was initiated in the early 1960s and is recognized around the world.[2] Its applicability and validity for almost every health discipline is the reason for its continued use today. During assessment of the health and physical status of patients, this system helps determine whether or not nitrous oxide/oxygen (N_2O/O_2) sedation is the best pain/anxiety management option.

B. The ASA established the following parameters for this classification system.

　1. ASA I—Normally healthy individuals who pose no risk to inhalation sedation. These patients are able to tolerate mild physical exertion and psychologic stresses. They do not possess any organic, physiologic, biochemical, or psychiatric disturbances.

　2. ASA II—Patients with mild-to-moderate systemic disease who, upon mild physical exertion and/or psychologic stress, are less tolerant than normal individuals. Fatigue and/or distress are factors that limit function in these individuals. Typically, patients with controlled and monitored health conditions, as well as those over age 65 or smokers, are classified as ASA II. Depending on their particular situation, these patients usually pose no risk to inhalation sedation.

　3. ASA III—Patients with severe systemic disease that limits but does not incapacitate activity are in this category. These patients cannot tolerate exertion and stress. Medical

consultation is recommended for these patients, particularly those with unstable conditions. These patients present greater risk for treatment; however, using N_2O/O_2 sedation does lessen anxiety and provide O_2 enrichment to the body systems.

4. ASA IV—Patients with severe systemic disease that limits activity and threatens life are not usually seen in an ambulatory health setting. Because of their unstable health problems, they are categorized as high risk for many situations; the potential for an acute emergency situation is great. Seek medical consultation and/or referral. N_2O/O_2 is usually not indicated except in emergency situations.

5. ASA V—The moribund patient who is not expected to survive more than 24 hours is listed as ASA V. In some cases, N_2O/O_2 is recommended for pain and anxiety relief in these final stages. The physiologic effects associated with chronic exposure to N_2O are of no importance here.

6. ASA VI—The patient in this classification is clinically dead but being maintained for organ harvest. There is no indication for N_2O/O_2 sedation.

III. *Assessing and Monitoring Vital Signs*

A. Significance

1. Obtaining preoperative, intraoperative, and postoperative vital signs are considered standards of care by the ASA and several other professional health societies and organizations.[3] They should be recorded in the patient's file at the initial visit and updated periodically thereafter.

2. Depending on the discipline, specialties with established guidelines for delivering anesthesia and sedation may recommend that vital signs be taken whenever N_2O/O_2 is used,[4-6] and state governing bodies may require that vital signs be taken.[7]

B. Number

1. There are a total of six vital signs: height, weight, body temperature, blood pressure, pulse, and respiration.

2. Blood pressure, pulse, and respiration are the most dynamic vital signs and are often recorded at each visit.

C. Vital signs recommended for N_2O/O_2 sedation

1. Blood pressure, pulse, and respiration should be obtained preoperatively to provide a baseline reference before N_2O/O_2 administration.

2. Intraoperative monitoring of vital signs is highly recommended during N_2O/O_2 sedation.

   a. Malamed[8] recommends monitoring blood pressure and pulse every 15 minutes for all patients and continuous pulse monitoring for children.

   b. Respiration can be monitored in several ways. A pretracheal stethoscope may be placed over the patient's trachea as a means of listening for air sounds.[8] A great advantage of N_2O/O_2 delivery is the reservoir bag. This serves as a supplemental supply of O_2 for the patient but also is a valid method of monitoring a patient's respiration. The bag mimics respiratory excursions, allowing the practitioner to monitor the frequency and depth of respirations with a reliable visual source. Cyanosis is not a reliable method for respiratory monitoring because it is apparent only long after distress has occurred.

3. Postoperative vital signs serve as a measure of recovery from N_2O/O_2 sedation. These values are compared with those obtained preoperatively and are assessed for the degree of variation. Details about recovery from N_2O/O_2 sedation are found in Chapter 15.

REFERENCES

1. Wolfe S: The practical approach to painless dentistry, *Dentistry Today,* 11:30-36, 1992.

2. American Society of Anesthesiologists: New classification of physical status, *Anesthesiology* 24:111, 1963.

3. Standards for basic intraoperative monitoring, *ASA Newsletter* 50:13, 1986.

4. American Association of Oral and Maxillofacial Surgeons, Committee on Anesthesia: *Office anesthesia evaluation manual,* ed 4, Rosemont, Ill, 1991, The Association.

5. Guidelines for the elective use of conscious sedation, deep sedation, and general anesthesia in pediatric patients, *Pediatrics* 76:317-321, 1985.

6. American Academy of Periodontology: Subcommittee on Anxiety and Pain Control of the Pharmacotherapeutics Committee: *Guidelines for the use of conscious sedation in periodontics,* Chicago, 1990, The Association.

7. American Dental Association, Council on Dental Education and Licensure: *Guidelines for the use of conscious sedation, deep sedation, and general anesthesia for dentists,* October 1996, American Dental Association.

8. Malamed SF: *Sedation: a guide to patient management,* ed 3, St Louis, 1995, Mosby.

9

Physical Properties and Pharmacokinetics of Nitrous Oxide

The conscientious healthcare provider offering nitrous oxide/oxygen (N₂O/O₂) sedation to patients must be knowledgeable about the actions of the drug. N₂O has many favorable attributes. Several of these characteristics relate to the pharmacologic properties of the drug and are particularly advantageous when using N₂O for general anesthesia; however, the same principles prove noteworthy in the ambulatory setting. While there is disagreement about whether N₂O deserves the "ideal" label, many agree that its role in healthcare is fundamental.

I. Physical/Chemical Properties of N_2O

A. N_2O is a stable, linear compound that is chemically diagramed as N≡N=O. It is a sweet-smelling, colorless gas.

B. The boiling point of N_2O, which is $-88.5°$ C ($-127°$ F), indicates that it is a gas at room temperature. When compressed into a cylinder, N_2O becomes a liquid.

C. The substance itself is nonflammable; however, N_2O supports combustion. If the gas comes in contact with a substance or flame of $1200°$ F, decomposition of the gas will occur. If the decomposition occurs at high temperature and elevated pressure (inside a cylinder or high-pressure pipeline), a violent chemical reaction such as an explosion will occur. If N_2O is present near an open flame the flame will burn brighter.[1]

D. Because N_2O like O_2 is an oxidizing gas, no hydrocarbon substances such as lubricants, grease, or oil should be used on any N_2O storage, distribution, or dispensing equipment. Of particular concern is the operation of such equipment in a manner that will increase the temperature of the N_2O. The most common example is the quick opening of valves, which causes a rapid pressure increase. The phenomenon known as the *heat of compression* can increase the gas temperature to a level that will ignite any hydrocarbon contaminants and cause a chemical reaction resulting in fire or explosion. This reaction could occur with any inorganic contaminant acting as a fuel.

E. The molecular weight of N_2O is 44. Its specific gravity is 1.53, which indicates that it is heavier than air (gr = 1) or pure O_2 (gr = 1.15).

F. N_2O is found in minimal concentrations (6 ppm) in the atmosphere.[2] Anesthetic N_2O contributes approximately 1% of the total amount.[3] As ultraviolet light combines with N_2O and O_2, free radicals (i.e., nitric oxide) are produced, which can affect the ozone.[4] Several natural and man-made methods release N_2O into the atmosphere (i.e., decomposition of pine wood).

II. Physical/Chemical Properties of O_2

A. Preparation
   1. O_2 is primarily prepared by fractional evaporation of liquid air.
   2. Air is cooled and compressed until it liquefies. O_2 compresses to a pale blue liquid at $-183°$ C.
   3. Nitrogen (N) and other elements evaporate, leaving liquid O_2.

B. Characteristics
   1. In a gaseous state O_2 is odorless, colorless, and tasteless.
   2. It makes up approximately 21% of the earth's atmosphere.
   3. The molecular weight of O_2 is 32; its specific gravity is 1.105 (air = 1).
   4. Like N_2O, O_2 supports combustion but is not itself flammable. It will react similarly to N_2O when it contacts a combustible material.
   5. O_2 is compressed gas in cylinders. The dial in the regulator gauge will accurately depict the O_2 content in the cylinder. As the gas is consumed, the dial will drop proportionally.

C. Uses
   1. There are several uses for O_2. The steel industry is one of the largest consumers of O_2.
   2. O_2 is the required co-component of N_2O when N_2O is being used for sedation. Current sedation equipment described in this text guarantees a minimum O_2 delivery of 30% to provide at least the amount that is found naturally in air.

III. *Pharmacokinetic Properties of N_2O*

A. Pharmacokinetic aspects of a drug affect its uptake, distribution, metabolism, and elimination in the body. Inhaled agents such as N_2O express their actions on the body by moving across partial pressure gradients. The agent will move from a higher- to a lower-pressure gradient. Uptake, distribution, and ultimately the onset and recovery of anesthesia depend on the solubility and potency of the drug. The interaction between a drug, the brain, and other tissues until equilibrium is reached is expressed in values called partition coefficients. These values indicate the ease or difficulty of drug transfer to the brain and body.

1. The difference between the partial pressures of a gas (N_2O) and a liquid (blood) indicates how easily the agent will cross the pulmonary membrane and enter the bloodstream. This is called the *blood/gas partition coefficient.* The solubility of the drug then determines how much is needed to reach the brain to begin clinical actions.

   a. If a drug is highly soluble it will diffuse immediately into the blood and be distributed throughout the body. Its blood/gas partition coefficient will be high, indicating that a large quantity of drug will be necessary to achieve the blood level required for movement of the agent to the brain. Therefore it will take a large quantity of drug and a longer time period before clinical effects are evident.

   b. If a drug is relatively insoluble, only small quantities will be necessary to achieve equilibrium. Onset of clinical action will be rapid. Also, the concentration of the molecules in the alveoli will be high.

   c. N_2O is an example of a poorly soluble or relatively insoluble drug. Its blood/gas partition coefficient is 0.47. It remains unchanged in the blood; the O_2 component is not available for use in the body because N_2O does not break down. Uptake by the body is limited, indicating that only a small quantity of N_2O is necessary to reach the required blood concentration. Therefore peak clinical effects may be seen within 3 to 5 minutes after initiation of the agent (Figure 9-1).

   d. There is a major difference in partial pressure gradients between N_2O and N. N_2O is approximately 34 times greater than N (Figure 9-2). Because of this, N_2O will rapidly replace the N occupying any body space. Not only will N_2O physically replace it, but it will also increase the volume and/or pressure of that space depending on its rigid vs. nonrigid confines. Specific conditions regarding this phenomenon are described in Chapter 10.

2. Other partition coefficients of N_2O and tissues, muscles, and fat are low. Equilibration occurs quickly in these instances because of the inability of most tissues to hold

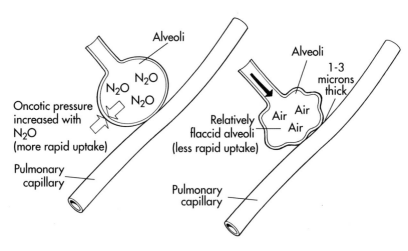

Figure 9-1   Effects of gas solubility.

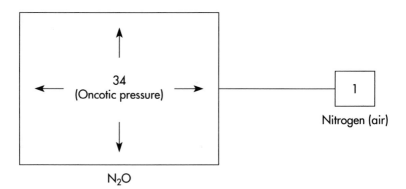

Figure 9-2   Expansion of N_2O molecules in air spaces.

N_2O. Because of this, N_2O is not stored in the body to any extent; thus elimination is not impeded.[5]

B. Eger introduced the concentration effect (Figure 9-3) of N_2O upon induction.[6] The concentration effect occurs when high concentrations of N_2O are delivered to the patient ($>70\%$ N_2O). These concentrations are delivered during general anesthesia.

   1. At high concentrations, alveolar partial pressures are reached rapidly and there is little decrease in the concentration of the gas. In addition, when delivering these high concentrations of N_2O, the volume of inspired gas is increased. Negative pressure is produced, drawing more gas into the lungs and increasing the volume.

   2. At lower concentrations the concentration effect is not significant. When administering analgesic percentages of N_2O, the rate of uptake is not affected.

C. As high concentrations of N_2O promote the rapid uptake of the gas, there is a simultaneous effect occurring with the other gases being administered. The rapid uptake of N_2O allows the second gas to be drawn in much faster than it

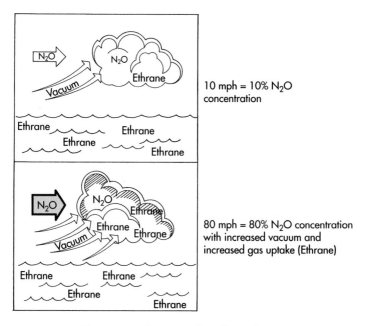

10 mph = 10% N_2O concentration

80 mph = 80% N_2O concentration with increased vacuum and increased gas uptake (Ethrane)

Figure 9-3   Concentration effect of N_2O.

would normally if it were being administered alone. This phenomenon, the second-gas effect (Figure 9-4), allows minimal amounts of a more potent anesthetic to be administered simultaneously with N_2O.[6]

D. N_2O is not metabolized through the liver. Ninety-nine percent of it is eliminated through the lungs without significant biotransformation in the body.[7] A miniscule (0.004%) amount of N_2O metabolizes in the gastrointestinal tract. Reduction occurs by the anaerobic bacteria *Pseudomonas* and produces potentially toxic-free radicals.[8,9] This process does not pose any significant threat to the body systems.

E. N_2O is difficult to use at extreme altitudes (i.e., above 10,000 feet). Because of the barometric pressure change, air ambulances and those administering N_2O/O_2 sedation at significant elevations must be aware of the need for a slight increase in N_2O concentration to obtain the same effects as at sea level.[10] In Denver (i.e., 5280 feet) for example, a 5% increase in N_2O may be necessary as compared with a location at sea level.

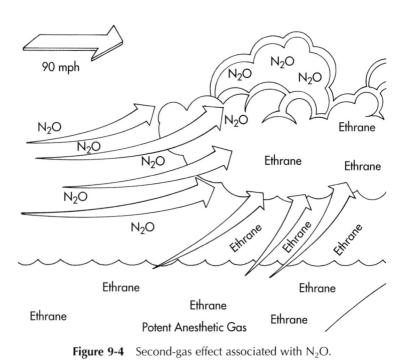

Figure 9-4   Second-gas effect associated with N_2O.

IV. *Potency of Anesthetic Agents*

A. The potency of an anesthetic agent indicates how strong or powerful the drug is or how effective it is at producing anesthesia. There are many potent drugs available for general anesthesia.

  1. N_2O is the weakest of all inhalation general anesthetics. However, nitrous oxide can produce general anesthesia.

  2. Drug potency is determined by assessing the minimum alveolar concentration (MAC) necessary to prevent movement in 50% of subjects responding to surgical incision.[11]

  3. The MAC for N_2O is 104% to 105%. This value indicates that at normal atmospheric pressure N_2O alone would not be able to produce profound surgical anesthesia. Hyperbaric conditions would have to exist for this to occur.[12]

  4. The MAC value and limited potency of N_2O add tremendously to its safety. Other anesthetic agents and their corresponding MAC values are listed in Box 9-1.

B. Halothane, isoflurane, enflurane, methoxyflurane, desflurane, and sevoflurane are examples of more potent inhalation agents used for general anesthesia. While their benefits are many, they also possess several negative factors, including toxicity, biotransformation, solubility, general complication issues, and negative effects on organ systems.

C. However, because of the second-gas effect from N_2O, profound anesthesia is produced using decreased concentrations of the drugs while reducing the potential for negative side effects.

BOX 9-1
Minimum Alveolar Concentration (MAC)
Values for Inhalation Anesthetics

Desflurane	4.6%
Enflurane	1.6%
Halothane	.75%
Isoflurane	1.2%
Methoxyflurane	.16%
Nitrous Oxide	104%
Sevoflurane	1.7%

V. Toxicity

A. When N_2O is used on healthy patients for clinical procedures of reasonable length, toxicity is insignificant or nonexistent. The effects of N_2O on body systems are discussed in Chapter 10.

B. Research studies done with both animals and humans indicate that prolonged exposure to N_2O can have a negative effect on vitamin B_{12} and its role in DNA synthesis. As vitamin B_{12} is inactivated its dependent enzyme, methionine synthase, is inhibited, resulting in bone marrow depression. Further discussion of the effects associated with prolonged N_2O exposure is found in Chapters 16 and 17.

REFERENCES

1. Fettes, WC: Personal communication, August 1996.
2. Maskell K, Mintzer IM, Callander BA: Basic science of climate change, *Lancet* 342:1027-1031, 1993.
3. Sherman SJ, Cullen BF: Nitrous oxide and the greenhouse effect, *Anesthesiology* 68:816-817, 1988.
4. Dale O, Husum B: Nitrous oxide: a threat to personnel and global environment? *Acta Anaesthesiol Scand* 38:777-779, 1994.
5. Eger EI II: Pharmacokinetics. In Eger EI II, editor: *Nitrous oxide N_2O,* New York, 1985, Elsevier Science Publishing.
6. Eger EI II: Uptake and distribution. In Miller RD, editor: *Anesthesia,* ed 4, vol 1, New York, 1994, Churchill Livingstone.
7. Stoelting RD: *Pharmacology and physiology in anesthetic practice,* ed 2, Philadelphia, 1991, JB Lippincott.
8. Hong K et al: Metabolism of nitrous oxide by human and rat intestinal contents, *Anesthesiology* 52:16-19, 1980.
9. Hong K et al: Biotransformation of nitrous oxide, *Anesthesiology* 53:354-355, 1980.
10. Stoelting RD: *Pharmacology and physiology in anesthetic practice,* ed 2, Philadelphia, 1991, JB Lippincott.
11. Eger EI II, Saidman LJ, Brandstater B: Minimum alveolar anesthetic concentration: a standard of anesthetic potency, *Anesthesiology* 26:756, 1965.
12. Eger EI II: MAC. In Eger EI II, editor: *Nitrous oxide N_2O,* New York, 1985, Elsevier Science Publishing.

SUGGESTED READINGS

Cullen DJ: Anesthetic pharmacology and critical care, *Acute Care* 14-15:3-25, 1988-89.

Dale O, Brown JR Jr: Clinical pharmacokinetics of the inhalational anaesthetics, *Clinical pharmacokinetics,* 12:145-167, 1987.

Hardman JG, Limbird LE, editors: *Goodman and Gillman's: the pharmacologic basis of therapeutics,* ed 9, New York, 1996, McGraw-Hill.

Joyce JL: Inhalation anesthetics, *AORN Journal* 52:77-83, 1990.

Longnecker DE, Miller FL: Pharmacology of inhalation anesthetics. In Rogers M et al, editors: *Principles and practice of anesthesiology,* St Louis, 1993, Mosby.

Stenqvist O: Nitrous oxide kinetics, *Acta Anaesthesiol Scand* 38:757-760, 1994.

Stoelting RD: *Pharmacology and physiology in anesthetic practice,* ed 2, Philadelphia, 1991, JB Lippincott.

10

Nitrous Oxide Interaction with the Body

The scientific study of nitrous oxide (N_2O) and its effect on the human body began with Horace Wells and has continued ever since. The literature is deluged with articles covering virtually every possible aspect of the drug. N_2O is an inhalant anesthetic drug, and its interaction with the body is compared with that of other inhalation anesthetics such as halothane, isoflurane, and enflurane. The debate as to whether N_2O is a friend or foe to the human body has been interesting to follow. Dr. Edmond Eger II, one of the most notable experts in the world on the subject, has had varying opinions on the virtues of N_2O. However, in a recent study Eger et al[1] examined several controversial aspects of the effects of N_2O and concluded that continued use of N_2O should be supported. Healthcare professionals should always encourage further scientific questioning and study.

I. N_2O Interaction with Body Systems and Conditions

A. Cardiovascular system

1. N_2O does not negatively affect the cardiovascular system to produce any *significant* physiologic changes. The interaction of several cardiovascular functions such as contractility, output, stroke volume, heart rate, and arrhythmias with N_2O have been researched in the past.[1-5]

2. N_2O effects on cardiac output differ in the literature. Slight increases have been noted as well as mild decreases. Dosage and the sympathomimetic effects of the drug may account for subtle differences.[1-5]

3. Blood flow to major organs is not significantly affected.[3]

4. N_2O with oxygen (O_2) does not create adverse cardiovascular conditions. Conversely, it has a positive effect on myocardial ischemia by providing supplemental O_2 and can be helpful in myocardial infarction.[6,7]

5. Blood pressure effects from N_2O may be dose related. In most instances blood pressure will not be affected by the N_2O concentrations commonly used in ambulatory settings. Eger et al[1] found blood pressure readings to be lower when N_2O/O_2 was used.

6. N_2O/O_2 sedation does not pose any significant negative effect on the cardiovascular system and can therefore be used with common conditions such as:
   a. Atherosclerosis/arteriosclerosis
   b. Rheumatic fever/heart murmur/congenital conditions
   c. Angina pectoris/myocardial infarction
   d. Surgery (valve, pacemaker, bypass, transplant)
   e. Hypertension
   f. Bleeding diathesis

B. Central nervous system (CNS)
   1. N_2O, like other anesthetics, has the ability to depress the CNS; however, the exact mechanism is unknown.[4]
   2. Comparatively, N_2O's effect on cerebral blood flow, intracranial pressure, and O_2 consumption appears to be less significant than that of other inhaled anesthetics.[4,8]
   3. The dosage of N_2O has an effect on the frequency and voltage changes on electroencephalograms (EEGs).[4,8]
   4. Because of the rapid replacement of nitrogen (N_2) with N_2O in air spaces, notable intracranial pressure increases were found in cases of pneumoencephalography. N_2O should not be used for 1 week after this procedure.[8]
   5. Evidence of injury to the nervous system has been shown in cases of chronic exposure to N_2O. Numbness and weakness in the extremities are seen as symptoms, as is ataxic gait.[2] This subject is discussed in detail in Chapter 16.
   6. N_2O/O_2 sedation does not pose any significant negative effect on the CNS, and therefore can be used with common conditions such as:
   a. Cerebrovascular accident (stroke)
   b. Seizure disorder/fainting spells
   c. Parkinson's disease

C. Respiratory system
   1. Upper respiratory tract infections or conditions commonly compromise air exchange through the nose. If the patient is unable to breathe through his/her nose, insufficient amounts of N_2O/O_2 will enter the respiratory system.

a. Any type of common infection leading to a cold, cough, sinus infection, bronchitis, allergy-related symptoms, etc. may occlude the nasal passages such that adequate air exchange at the alveolar level will be incomplete.

b. Additionally, if N_2O/O_2 is elected to be used for an individual with mild symptoms, the drying effect of the gases may create mucous plugs and negatively affect the pulmonary tree. Again, sedation may be incomplete and inadequate.

c. Sinus cavities represent rigid, noncompliant air spaces. The nonexpansive nature of these areas leads to an increase in pressure when N_2O is administered. When sinusitis is present, the additional pressure may be uncomfortable for the patient.

d. Contamination and disease transmission are potential complications associated with upper respiratory tract infections, tuberculosis infections, and HIV/AIDS. Because of the possibility of their transmission, it is recommended to sterilize all conducting tubing, the reservoir bag, and the breathing apparatus or dispose of these materials.

2. Although rare in occurrence, silent regurgitation and concommitant aspiration remain controversial issues with regard to N_2O/O_2 sedation. The concern lies in whether pharyngeal/laryngeal reflexes remain unaffected during N_2O/O_2 sedation.[9]

a. Dye studies done with a 5- to 10-minute exposure to 50% N_2O were negative for aspiration[10]; no evidence of aspiration occurred in 25 children given N_2O concentrations between 20% and 65%.[11] A 30-minute N_2O exposure, however, revealed two aspirations in 10 volunteers.[12]

b. Most procedures performed in an ambulatory health setting are time intensive, and patients may not have fasted. Therefore the potential for positive aspiration resulting from silent regurgitation exists.

c. Because this is a potentially life-threatening situation, it is critical to use the appropriate titration technique when administering N_2O/O_2 sedation to avoid oversedation. Equally as critical is continuous monitoring of the patient.

3. Patients susceptible to hypoxia because of airway resistance, impaired function, or movement appear to be at a slight risk for N_2O/O_2 sedation. Eger[9] indicates that this may not be a significant issue.

a. Examples of conditions in this category are emphysema, chronic bronchitis, and asthma. There has never been a reported allergy to N_2O. Its use is not contraindicated for asthma patients because it is nonirritating to mucous membranes. In fact, the sedative nature of N_2O/O_2 has a positive influence on asthmatic patients because anxiety often triggers an asthmatic episode.

b. For patients chronically debilitated with other respiratory conditions, N_2O/O_2 may be considered a relative contraindication.

   i. Some of these patients may be on hypoxic drive. As carbon dioxide (CO_2) normally initiates respiration in healthy individuals, O_2 may be the stimulus for those compromised with chronic obstructive pulmonary diseases (COPD).

   ii. If so, choosing N_2O/O_2 sedation would be inappropriate because this modality provides supplemental O_2. The increased O_2 heightens the O_2 blood saturation level to a point at which the breathing stimulus is gone. Breathing could cease and hypoxia could result.

   iii. In the majority of cases, persons on hypoxic drive are very ill. Some will not be able to be treated in an ambulatory setting; most represent an ASA IV risk (see Chapter 8). Medical consultation is recommended before any treatment.

4. The condition of pneumothorax (air/gas in the pleural cavity) may be complicated with N_2O. The expansive quality of the gas causes increased expansion of the size of the pneumothorax. This condition demands medical attention. In general anesthesia, if 75% N_2O is delivered, the volume of the space could be increased up to 300%; its size could double within 10 minutes.[13] Even though in the ambulatory setting the doses of N_2O would be much smaller, the pharmacokinetic nature of the gas is constant. N_2O/O_2 sedation should be avoided in this situation.

5. Therefore N_2O/O_2 sedation presents the following recommendations regarding the respiratory system:

a. Emphysema—Physician discretion for hypoxic drive

b. Chronic bronchitis—Physician discretion for hypoxic drive

c. Tuberculosis—Dispose of contaminated items

d. HIV/AIDS—Dispose of contaminated items

   e. Upper respiratory tract infections—Postpone N_2O/O_2
    until resolved
   f. Pneumothorax—Postpone N_2O/O_2 until resolved

D. Hematopoietic system

  1. Megaloblastic bone marrow changes have been found in patients who have been exposed to high concentrations of N_2O for an extended period.[14] N_2O has been implicated in the interference of the vitamin B_{12}-dependent enzyme methionine synthase. This enzyme is necessary for DNA synthesis and erythrocyte production.[4,8]

  2. Another concern with hematopoietic conditions is the decrease in O_2 available to the body because of red blood cell deficiency, impairment, destruction, and/or other conditions affecting red blood cells. Inhalation sedation is often recommended because of the supplemental O_2 it delivers.[15]

  3. Therefore N_2O/O_2 sedation can be recommended for the following:

   a. Anemias
   b. Methemoglobinemia
   c. Sickle-cell anemia
   d. Leukemia
   e. Hemophilia
   f. Polycythemia vera

E. Endocrine system

  1. Inhalation sedation using N_2O/O_2 has no negative effect on the endocrine system.

  2. Therefore it poses no risk for individuals with any condition involving this system.

   a. Diabetes
   b. Thyroid gland dysfunction
   c. Adrenal dysfunction

F. Hepatic system

  1. N_2O is not metabolized in the liver, nor does it affect the liver in the presence of liver impairment.[1,16-18]

  2. Therefore N_2O/O_2 sedation does not pose any effect on the following conditions:

   a. Hepatitis
   b. Jaundice
   c. Other

G. Gastrointestinal system

  1. Because of the expansive nature of the gas and its propensity for insufflating air spaces within the body, N_2O diffuses into these areas much more rapidly than N_2 exits. The gas entering nonrigid-walled air spaces in the

body causes the spaces to expand. This expansion and possible pressure can be problematic.

2. The bowel exemplifies a nonrigid air space in which expansion occurs. If a patient presents with a bowel obstruction, it would be less desirable to use N_2O/O_2 sedation because the N_2O could affect the condition by increasing expansion, pressure, and discomfort.[19]

3. Therefore the following recommendations regarding the gastrointestinal system and N_2O/O_2 sedation are made:
   a. Ulcer—No negative effect using N_2O/O_2
   b. Obstructions—Postpone N_2O/O_2 until resolved

H. Genitourinary/reproductive systems

1. N_2O/O_2 sedation does not pose any negative effect on the genitourinary system itself. Any time disease transmissibility is an issue, proper infection control procedures and disposal of appropriate equipment are recommended.

2. Pregnancy is a normal physiologic state not to be confused with a disease state. Treatment considerations are important during organogenesis in the first trimester and when low O_2-tension levels are possible in the last trimester. Most pharmacologic agents cross the placental barrier; N_2O is no exception.
   a. It is necessary to maintain adequate O_2 levels to prevent spontaneous abortion. However, the O_2 fail-safe feature inherent in updated equipment prevents this occurrence.
   b. The N_2O/O_2 combination has been a commonly used pharmacologic agent in obstetrics for centuries. Research confirms its safety with pregnant women.[20] In case of pregnancy, the following items regarding N_2O/O_2 sedation in the ambulatory setting should be considered.
      i.   Obtain appropriate medical consultation before the use of any drug for the duration of the pregnancy.
      ii. Avoid N_2O during the first trimester. N_2O, when delivered appropriately, should not physiologically threaten the fetus; however, like radiation, N_2O/O_2 could be blamed unfairly by the psychologically affected mother should fetal anomalies manifest.
      iii. It is best to leave the decision whether to use N_2O/O_2 sedation for a pregnant woman up to the attending medical personnel.

3. Therefore regarding these body systems, recommendations for N_2O/O_2 sedation are:
   a. Kidney disease—No negative effect using N_2O/O_2

       b. Sexually transmitted diseases—Dispose of contaminated items

       c. Pregnancy—Medical consultation recommended

I. Neuromuscular system

   1. N_2O does not provide direct skeletal muscle relaxation. In higher concentrations, muscle rigidity can be seen with N_2O.[21]

   2. N_2O/O_2 has no effect on patients with neuromuscular conditions.

   3. Therefore the use of N_2O/O_2 sedation can be recommended with the following conditions involving the neuromusculature:

       a. Multiple sclerosis

       b. Muscular dystrophy

       c. Cerebral palsy

       d. Myasthenia gravis

J. Middle ear disturbances

   1. As N_2O infiltrates the rigid, noncompliant area of the middle ear, increased pressure results. Significant damage such as hearing loss, tympanic membrane rupture, graft displacement, and other complications have been observed.[22-25] Also, the negative pressure that results from the rapid departure of N_2O after general anesthesia can cause other injuries, especially after recent ear, nose, and throat complications.[26]

   2. Therefore careful consideration of N_2O/O_2 sedation should be applied with the following conditions:

       a. Middle ear disturbances—Postpone N_2O/O_2 sedation until resolved

       b. Recent ear, nose, throat infections—Medical consultation advised

K. Cancer

   1. N_2O does not combine with any of the formed blood elements, nor does it affect metastatic cells.[27]

   2. N_2O/O_2 has been used in the final stages of life as an adjuvant to other pharmacologic methods for pain and anxiety management. In these situations, the untoward effects caused by chronic exposure to N_2O are irrelevant.[28,29]

   3. Therefore N_2O/O_2 sedation can provide additional comfort for the following condition:

       a. Cancer—Positive analgesic effect in final stages of life

L. Mind-altering conditions

   1. Mind-altering conditions must be carefully considered before N_2O/O_2 administration.

2. If the patient is unable to understand the procedure and its effects, he/she may negatively perceive the associated signs and symptoms.

3. If the patient is suffering or recovering from addiction or mental illness, the relaxing, euphoric sensations may exacerbate or trigger unwanted episodes or encourage addictive behaviors. Discretion is warranted.

4. Therefore careful consideration should be taken regarding N_2O/O_2 sedation when the following conditions exist:
   a. Mental illness
   b. Mental retardation
   c. Autism
   d. Alzheimer's disease
   e. Chemical dependency, including alcoholism and substance abuse

M. Allergies
1. For more than 150 years there have been no known reported allergies to N_2O.
2. Therefore N_2O/O_2 sedation does not pose any effect on the following conditions:
   a. Allergies to drugs
   b. Seasonal allergies
   c. Miscellaneous allergies
3. Persons sensitive to latex may experience contact dermatitis when using the nasal hood. Placing a gauze barrier between the skin and nasal hood may alleviate this problem.

N. Malignant hyperthermia
1. This condition may unexpectedly occur as a result of an individual's response to certain drugs. Patients knowledgeable of familial tendencies and history can be tested to avoid this problem.
2. Because of the pharmacologic, pharmacokinetic, and benign nature of N_2O, inhalation sedation with N_2O/O_2 may be preferred over other methods.
3. Therefore the complications associated with malignant hyperthermia may be avoided with N_2O/O_2 sedation.

O. Nutritional disorders
1. N_2O/O_2 sedation does not affect any nutritional conditions.
2. Therefore it can safely be used should these conditions be present:
   a. High cholesterol level
   b. Eating disorders

II. N_2O Interaction with Medications

A. There is no direct interaction of N_2O with medications taken by the patient.[30]

B. N_2O may enhance drugs that are used directly to induce sleep or that list drowsiness as a side effect.

III. Additional Considerations Regarding N_2O/O_2 Use

A. Altered mental states or levels of consciousness indicate a situation warranting careful consideration before N_2O/O_2 administration.

1. N_2O/O_2 use should be avoided for a patient presenting himself/herself intoxicated from drugs or alcohol. Alcohol and barbiturates are classified as sedative-hypnotic drugs.

   a. Although alcohol has been historically prescribed and acknowledged as a mild anxiolytic, it is not a recommended method of sedation for a patient in an ambulatory health setting.

   b. Barbiturates are quite effective sedative agents when prescribed in a professional manner; however, patients prescribing their own drugs and dosages before their appointments should not be treated in these settings.

2. Patients under psychiatric and/or psychologic care should be carefully considered before N_2O/O_2 use. Many patients are treated with antidepressant or other psychotropic drugs. Drug interaction is not at issue in these cases, but rather the potentiality of exacerbating the negative aspects of the condition. Seek medical consultation before N_2O/O_2 administration.

3. For those professionals in emergency medicine, whether in the field or hospital, it is unwise to use N_2O/O_2 for anyone in shock, in a semiconscious state, or presenting with head/facial injuries. These patients, most likely, will not be able to self-administer the 50/50 N_2O/O_2 mixture using the demand-flow system.

4. Severely phobic individuals will not benefit by N_2O/O_2 administration. These persons should be in the care of a competent expert in the field. It is unlikely that N_2O/O_2

will be able to provide adequate relief to accomplish the intended procedure. It is likely that N_2O/O_2 will make the situation worse as the patient will resist the calming effects of the drug. Physical agitation and acts of aggression could result.

5. In some cases, patients with claustrophobic tendencies may feel uncomfortable using a nasal hood. Often these patients relax sufficiently during N_2O/O_2 sedation that this is not a problem.

B. When time is taken to explain the N_2O/O_2 procedure and words are carefully chosen to present the positive effects, most patients will consent. If a patient is unwilling or does not give consent, the practitioner must never force the continuance of the procedure. This would undoubtedly destroy any patient/operator trust and place the practitioner in legal jeopardy.

REFERENCES

1. Eger EI II et al: Clinical pharmacology of nitrous oxide: an argument for its continued use, *Anesth Anal* 71:575-585, 1990.
2. Eger EI II, Gaskey NJ: A review of the present status of nitrous oxide, *J Assoc Nurse Anes* 54:29-36, 1986.
3. Eisele JH Jr: Cardiovascular effects of nitrous oxide. In Eger EI II: *Nitrous oxide N_2O,* New York, 1985, Elsevier Science Publishing.
4. Stoelting RK: *Pharmacology and physiology in anesthetic practice,* ed 2, Philadelphia, 1991, JB Lippincott.
5. Stoelting RK, Miller RD: *Basics of anesthesia,* ed 2, New York, 1989, Churchill Livingstone.
6. Thompson PL, Lown B: Nitrous oxide as an analgesic in acute myocardial infarction, *J Am Med Assoc* 235:924-927, 1976.
7. Kerr F et al: Nitrous oxide analgesia in myocardial infarction, *Lancet* 1:63-66, 1972.
8. Frost EA: Central nervous system effects of nitrous oxide. In Eger EI II: *Nitrous oxide N_2O,* New York, 1985, Elsevier Science Publishing
9. Eger EI II: Respiratory effects of nitrous oxide. In Eger EI II: *Nitrous oxide N_2O,* New York, 1985, Elsevier Science Publishing.
10. Cleaton-Jones P: The laryngeal-closure reflex and nitrous oxide-oxygen anesthesia, *Anesthesiology* 45:569-570, 1976.
11. Roberts GJ, Wignall BK: Efficacy of the laryngeal reflex during oxygen-nitrous oxide sedation (relative analgesia), *Br J Anesth* 54:1277-1281, 1982.
12. Rubin J et al: Laryngeal incompetence during experimental "relative analgesia" using 50% nitrous oxide in children, *Anesthesiology* 49:1005-1007, 1977.
13. Eger EI II, Saidman LJ. Hazards of nitrous oxide anesthesia in bowel obstruction and pneumothorax, *Anesthesiology* 26:61-66. 1965.
14. Nunn JE: Clinical aspects of the interaction between nitrous oxide and vitamin B_{12}, *Br J Anesth* 59:3-13, 1987.
15. Malamed SF: Sedation: *A guide to patient management,* St Louis, 1995, Mosby.
16. Brodsky JB: Toxicity of nitrous oxide. In Eger EI II: *Nitrous oxide N_2O,* New York, 1985, Elsevier Science Publishing.

17. Lampe GJ et al: Nitrous oxide does not impair hepatic function on young or old surgical patients, *Anesth Analg* 71:606-609, 1990.

18. Longnecker DE, Miller FL: Pharmacology of inhalation anesthetics. In Rogers M et al, editors: *Principles and practice of anesthesiology,* St Louis, 1993, Mosby.

19. Eger EI II: Pharmacokinetics. In Eger EI II, editor: *Nitrous oxide N₂O,* New York, 1985, Elsevier Science Publishing.

20. Marx FG, Bassell GM: Nitrous oxide in obstetrics. In Eger EI II: *Nitrous oxide N₂O,* New York, 1985, Elsevier Science Publishing.

21. Miller RD: Neuromuscular effects of nitrous oxide. In Eger EI II: *Nitrous oxide N₂O,* New York, 1985, Elsevier Science Publishing.

22. Donlon JV Jr: Anesthesia and eye, ear, nose, and throat surgery. In Miller RD: *Anesthesia,* ed 4, New York, 1994, Churchill Livingstone.

23. Barash P, Cullen B, Stoelting R: *Clinical anesthesia,* ed 2, Philadelphia, 1992, JB Lippincott.

24. Mann MS, Woodsford PV, Jones RM: Anesthetic carrier gases, *Anesthesiology* 40:8-11, 1985.

25. Waun JE, Sweitzer RH, Hamilton WK: Effect of nitrous oxide on middle ear mechanics and hearing activity, *Anesthesiology* 28:846-850, 1967.

26. Ohryn M: Tympanic membrane rupture following general anesthesia with nitrous oxide: a case report, *J Am Assoc Nurse Anesth* 63:42-44, 1995.

27. Malamed SF: *Sedation: a guide to patient management,* St Louis, 1995, Mosby.

28. Fosburg MT, Crone RK: Nitrous oxide analgesia for refractory pain in the terminally ill, *J Am Med Assoc* 250:511-513, 1983.

29. Foley LM: The treatment of pain in the patient with cancer, *CA Cancer J Clin* 36:194-215, 1986.

30. Dale O, Brown BR Jr: Clinical pharmacokinetics of the inhalational anaesthetics, *Clin Pharmacokinet* 12:145-167, 1987.

11

Anatomy and Physiology of Respiration

Any method of inhalation sedation involves those structures associated with the inhalation and exhalation of air and the exchange of gases. To integrate the pharmacologic properties of nitrous oxide (N_2O) into a clinical setting, the basic principles of the anatomy and physiology of respiration should be reviewed.

I. Respiratory System Design and Function

A. The respiratory system is primarily designed to perform the function of exchanging gases—functionally carbon dioxide (CO_2) and oxygen (O_2)—across pulmonary/capillary membranes. The design of the system allows this function to be performed continuously and with minimal effort by the body.[1]

B. Respiration is driven automatically by the brainstem (medulla oblongata) and voluntarily by the cerebral cortex.[2]

II. Anatomy of the Upper Airway

A. Nose
   1. The respiratory functions of the nose are to warm the air to body temperature, humidify the air, and filter the air for foreign particles via nose hair and cilia.
   2. Because the nose is also the primary entrance of gases used during inhalation sedation, it is critical to the effectiveness of the procedure that a patient is able to breathe well. Anatomic conditions affecting air passage through the nose (e.g., a deviated septum) may interfere with N_2O/O_2 delivery.

B. Pharynx
   1. The pharynx is a cylindrical, muscular tube about 12 to 14 cm long.

2. It is divided into three sections (Figure 11-1): the naso-pharynx, oropharynx, and laryngopharynx.

    a. The nasopharynx is located behind the nasal cavity. The adenoids, tonsils, and openings to the eustachian tubes are found here. The soft palate separates the nasopharynx from the oropharynx.

    b. The oropharynx opens into the mouth and serves as the link between the nasopharynx and the laryngopharynx. It serves as an entrance to the larynx and esophagus. Its parameters are the soft palate and the epiglottis at the level of the hyoid bone. The epiglottis is connected by the medial glossoepiglottic fold and bilateral glossoepiglottic fold. These folds create a depression called the *valleculae.* Lateral to this central area on either side is a piriform recess. These recesses are the primary location for collecting foreign objects, thereby protecting the lower airway.

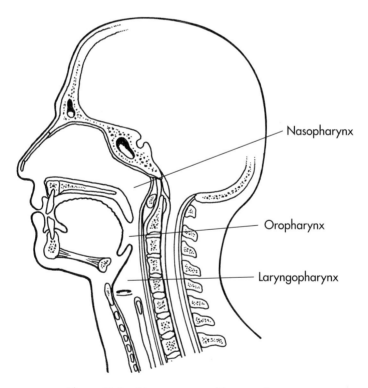

Nasopharynx

Oropharynx

Laryngopharynx

Figure 11-1   Naso-, oro-, and laryngopharynx.

c. The laryngopharynx begins at the epiglottis. The epiglottis is the cartilaginous, leaf-shaped structure that projects upward behind the tongue. This flaplike structure (Figure 11-2) directs material backward to the esophagus and prevents objects from entering the trachea during swallowing. The laryngopharynx extends from the epiglottis to the cricoid cartilage. The larynx lies inside the laryngopharnx. The framework of the laryngopharynx is made up of the thyroid cartilage, which is shaped like a shield, and the cricoid cartilage, which is shaped like a ring. Several muscle groups and ligaments cover these large structures. Both cartilages offer significant protection to the underlying larynx.

III. *Anatomy of the Lower Airway*

A. Larynx

1. The air passageway continues with the larynx. Pearl-colored vocal cords are housed here, which, when vibrated with air, produce vocal sound. The glottal opening at the vocal cords is the narrowest part of the entire airway.

2. The sensitive mucosa of the larynx is protected by strong muscles (false vocal cords), which adduct to prevent

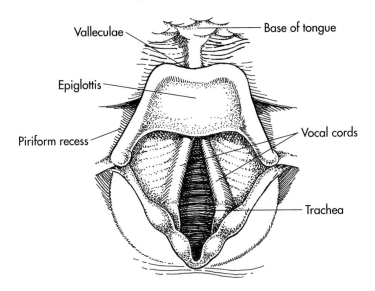

Figure 11-2   Larynx and epiglottis.

entry of foreign objects. If the larynx is irritated, the defensive cough reflex is initiated. Coughing occurs when high pressure is produced in the lower respiratory tract by the closing of the epiglottis and vocal cords and the contracting of expiratory and abdominal muscles. A sudden opening of the false vocal cords allows the air to explode out of the respiratory tract, carrying the foreign matter with it.[2] It is important to note that the use of N_2O for inhalation sedation allows this vital defensive reflex to remain intact.

B. Trachea

    1. The trachea, a muscular tube contiguous with the larynx, begins at the sixth cervical vertebrae and is surrounded by horseshoe-shaped cartilaginous rings. It is approximately 11 cm long with a lumen size of approximately 20 mm. Figure 11-3 shows the trachea and bronchi.

    2. The trachea bifurcates asymmetrically into the right and left bronchi. A highly sensitive, neurologically rich area, the carina (Figure 11-4), marks this bifurcation. The carina is considered a back-up defense mechanism for the cough reflex. If an object passes through the first defense site (larynx), the carina will cause the defensive cough to continue. Submucosal swelling and partial obstruction in this area can result from a strong stimulus and lead to asphyxiation.

C. Bronchi

    1. The right bronchus is approximately 2.5 cm long and deviates slightly from the trachea at approximately 25 degrees. Because of the minimal divergence from the trachea, aspirated foreign objects are commonly found in the right lung. Comparatively, the left bronchus is twice as long and smaller in diameter than its right counterpart. It deviates closer to 45 degrees from the trachea (see Figure 11-4).

    2. The main stem bronchi diverge into smaller branches responsible for the upper, middle, and lower lobes of the lung. The right bronchus divides into three branches, which link to three upper lobes, two middle lobes, and five lower lobes. The left bronchus bifurcates into two branches that give rise to five upper lobes and four lower lobes. Each lobe contains conducting and respiratory bronchioli with dependent alveolar ducts, sacs, and alveoli.

D. Bronchioles

    1. Bronchioles are a continued division of the bronchi but are identified by the lack of cartilage.

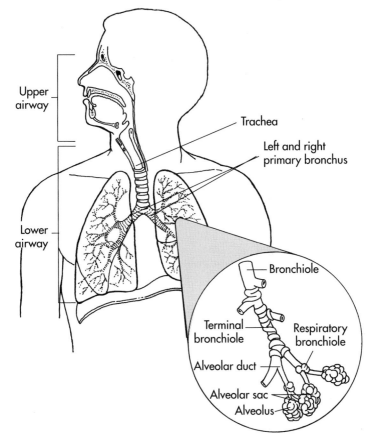

Figure 11-3 Trachea and bronchi.

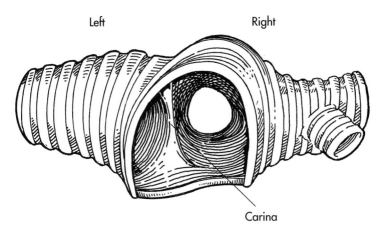

Figure 11-4 Carina located at the bifurcation of the bronchi.

2. The first 16 of the 23 generations of airways are considered conducting airways in normal anatomy.[2] These airways are incapable of exchanging gases. At generation 17 the respiratory bronchioli begin the respiratory zone. These are smaller than the parent bronchiolus but contain significantly more surface area.[2]

IV. Anatomy of the Respiratory Zone

A. Bronchioli, alveolar ducts, alveolar sacs, and alveoli
   1. Alveolar ducts mark the transition between bronchioli, alveolar sacs, and alveoli, as shown in Figure 11-3.
   2. Alveolar sacs "pouch" to form the thin-walled alveoli.
   3. It is in the 300 million alveoli of an adult that the exchange between air and blood takes place.[2]

V. Physiology of the Respiratory Mechanism

A. The medullary center in the brainstem controls the automatic respiratory process of breathing. Active inspiration is accomplished principally by the diaphragm and external intercostal muscles and assisted by the scalenes and sternomastoids. As the diaphragm moves downward, the chest wall expands, creating negative pressure in the pleural space, thereby allowing a vacuum effect to pull air into the system. This motion, producing a drop in air pressure in the lungs, provides the principal mechanics for inspiration.

B. Air continues to flow until pressures from inside the lung are equivalent to atmospheric pressure. Expiration occurs passively as the chest wall and lungs recoil. This recoil causes another pressure change in which the compressed air is quietly pushed out of the lungs. Expiration becomes active only when changes in respiratory demands such as exercise, abnormalities, or disease occur. This automatic, regular ebb-and-flow movement of air is called *tidal flow* because of its similarities to that of the ocean tide.[2]

C. Because of the pressure gradient that exists between the lung walls and the thoracic cavity, the lungs are distended and fill the cavity while atmospheric pressure pushes the chest wall inward. The fluid between the structures prevents the two from separating. If air enters the pleural cavity, as in a trauma, a pneumothorax results. The fluid holding the lungs against the wall cannot hold the two together.

D. The amount of gas inspired into the lungs (tidal volume) depends largely on the physical characteristics of the individual. Larger bodies hold more volume than smaller bodies; athletes have greater lung capacity than those with debilitating diseases; and males' lung volumes are approximately 25% greater than those of females.[3]

   1. In a normal-size adult of average physical ability and without lung disease, the tidal volume approaches 500 ml. *Minute ventilation* (volume) is the amount of gas brought into the lungs each minute. It is calculated by multiplying the tidal volume with the rate of respiration (eg., 500 ml $\times$ 12 $-$ 15 resp/min = approximately 6 to 7 L per minute).[1-3]

   2. Minute ventilation is significant in terms of N_2O administration because it deals with how much gas mixture ($N_2O + O_2$) should be given to a patient. Inadequate amounts are likely to produce a suffocating feeling and make the act of breathing laborious. Conversely, too much gas forced into the nasal hood of the delivery system will be wasted. Because it is not being consumed by the patient it will escape. This excess airflow not only blows into the patient's eyes, causing dryness, but also exposes personnel to unnecessary amounts of trace gas.

   3. *Alveolar ventilation* is the amount of air per minute entering the alveolar units capable of gas/blood exchange. This volume is less than the minute volume because not all of the inspired air reaches the alveoli during inspiration. A portion of the inhaled air occupies the conducting airways not able to participate in the gas/blood exchange, which are the nose, pharynx, trachea, and bronchi. This is known as *anatomic dead space.* Therefore alveolar ventilation is calculated by subtracting the dead space volume (approximately 150 ml) from the tidal volume and then multiplying by the respiration rate.[3]

E. The critical gas exchange from alveolus to capillary and vice versa occurs through simple diffusion across partial-pressure gradients.

   1. Atmospheric air is composed of 79% nitrogen (N_2), 21% O_2, and 0.04% CO_2. Other gases are negligible. Combined, these gases produce a pressure of 760 mm Hg at sea level. Because each component exerts the same amount of pressure, the concentration of each gas determines the amount of pressure exerted. This individual pressure is known as *partial pressure.*

2. A gas dissolved in blood also has a partial pressure. The amount of gas capable of dissolving in blood will depend on its solubility and partial pressure. Gases will always move from higher to lower pressure.[3]

3. The rate at which gases are exchanged depends primarily on the difference between partial pressures. If the gas entering the alveolus has a significantly higher partial pressure than that in the capillary, the gas explodes into the blood. This will occur until the partial pressure in the blood equals that of the alveoli.

   a. When N_2O/O_2 is administered, high concentrations of these gases are found in the alveolus, creating a high partial pressure. The capillary, possessing no N_2O originally, is quickly filled.

   b. N_2O is not readily absorbed by the blood. Because of this insolubility very little gas is absorbed into blood elements. Within minutes equilibrium between the partial pressures of the alveolus and capillary is achieved. This quick action continues as the gas-filled blood is carried to the brain; the onset of clinical symptoms is rapid once the gas reaches the brain.

   c. The converse of rapid infusion to the blood is also true. As the N_2O flow is terminated, capillary tension quickly rises to that above alveolar pressure. N_2O is quickly forced into the alveoli and exhaled through the lungs. Trace amounts of N_2O are metabolized in the body; however, the vast majority is removed rapidly through the lungs. During this process, N_2O exits faster than the nitrogen (N_2) that replaces it, thereby diluting the supply of O_2 and reducing the O_2 blood saturation (SaO_2). This phenomenon is called *diffusion hypoxia.*

   d. O_2 saturation levels are considered normal at 95% or above. Moderate hypoxemia occurs between 75% and 90%, while severe hypoxemia is categorized at levels below 75%.[4]

      i. A pulse oximeter is an instrument used to accurately measure O_2 saturation levels in the circulating blood. A small device is attached by a clip or adhesive to the patient's finger as shown in Figure 11-5. A light source passes through the blood, interpreting O_2 saturation through light absorption. See Appendix A for references.

      ii. While use of a pulse oximeter is not mandated to monitor O_2 saturation, it nonetheless reflects O_2 uptake at the cellular level. Therefore it can be

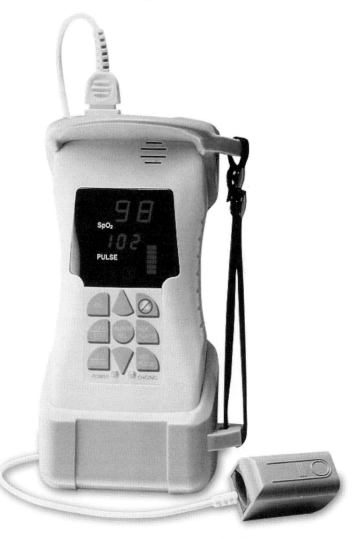

Figure 11-5   Pulse oximeter and digital sensor.

useful in detecting potential problems with O_2 administration.

iii. Consideration for the use of a pulse oximeter may be predicated on the advantages of simultaneously obtaining pulse rate and O_2 saturation levels. In addition, a record of calculated values may be printed and used for documentation in the patient's file.

F. Diffusion hypoxia
1. It has been hypothesized that headache, lethargy, and nausea can occur because of decreased O_2 saturation levels in the blood caused by the rapid exit of N_2O upon its termination. The application of 100% pure O_2 for the first 3 to 5 minutes after N_2O termination has been traditionally advocated to prevent O_2 desaturation of blood.
2. Researchers question the clinical significance of diffusion hypoxia and whether these symptoms are even associated. Quarnstrom et al[5] evaluated 104 patients and found no drop in SaO_2. He questions the necessity for postoperative O_2. Papageorge, Noonan, and Rosenberg[6] monitored 80 patients and found O_2 decreases to have a mean of 2.1%. In this study all O_2 decreases stabilized independently within 12 seconds to 15 minutes. Dunn-Russell et al[7] assessed 24 children who were allowed to breathe room air after N_2O/O_2 sedation. None exhibited abnormal SaO_2 levels or exhibited any of the associated side effects. Murphy and Splinter[8] claimed the same conclusion with children undergoing general anesthesia. Brodsky et al[9] observed only 3 of 60 patients with SaO_2 decreases. Hovagim et al[10] states that even though postoperative O_2 is given, there may be mild decreases in O_2 saturation.
3. Even though researchers claim diffusion hypoxia is not clinically significant, there are still patients who face postoperative headache, lethargy, and nausea. Administering 100% O_2 postoperatively for a minimum of 3 to 5 minutes prevents these symptoms from occurring. Lampe et al[11] agree that it continues to be prudent practice to deliver postoxygenation. As authors and clinicians we concur.

REFERENCES

1. Light RW: Mechanics of respiration. In George RB et al, editors: *Chest medicine: essentials of pulmonary and critical care medicine,* Baltimore, 1995, Williams & Wilkins.
2. George RB, Chesson AL, Rennard SI: Functional anatomy of the respiratory system. In George RB et al, editors: *Chest medicine: essentials of pulmonary and critical care medicine, Baltimore,* 1995, Williams & Wilkins.
3. Stoelting RD: *Pharmacology and physiology in anesthestic practice,* ed 2, Philadelphia, 1991, JB Lippincott.
4. Shapiro BA: *Oxygenation: measurement and clinical assessment,* Philadelphia, 1979, JB Lippincott.
5. Quarnstrom FC et al: Clinical study of diffusion hypoxia after nitrous oxide analgesia, *Anesth Prog* 38:21-23, 1991.

6. Papageorge MB, Noonan LW Jr, Rosenberg M: Diffusion hypoxia: another view, *Anesth Pain Control Dent* 2:143-149, 1993.

7. Dunn-Russell T et al: Oxygen saturation and diffusion hypoxia in children following nitrous oxide sedation, *Pediatr Dent* 16:88-92, 1993.

8. Murphy IL, Splinter WM: The clinical significance of diffusion hypoxia in children, *Can J Anaesth* 37:S40, 1990.

9. Brodsky JB et al: Diffusion hypoxia: a reappraisal using pulse oximetry, *J Clin Mon* 4:244-246, 1988.

10. Hovagim AR et al: Arterial oxygen desaturation in adult dental patients receiving conscious sedation, *J Oral Maxillofac Surg* 47:936-939, 1989.

11. Lampe GH et al: Postoperative hypoxemia after nonabdominal surgery: a frequent event not caused by nitrous oxide, *Anesth Analg* 71:597-601, 1990.

SUGGESTED READINGS

Artru AA: Survival time during hypoxia: effects of nitrous oxide, thiopental, and hypothermia, *Anesth Analg* 67:913-916, 1988.

Eger EI II: Respiratory effects of nitrous oxide. In Eger EI II: *Nitrous oxide N₂O,* New York, 1985, Elsevier Science Publishing.

Mueller WA et al: Pulse oximetry monitoring of sedated pediatric dental patients, *Anesth Prog* 32:237-240, 1985.

Papageorge MB et al: Supplemental oxygen after outpatient oral and maxillofacial surgery, *Anesth Prog* 39:24-27, 1993.

12

Titration of Nitrous Oxide/Oxygen Gases

Titration is a method of administering a substance by adding definitive amounts of a drug until an endpoint is reached. For nitrous oxide/oxygen (N_2O/O_2) sedation, N_2O is given in incremental doses until a patient has reached a comfortable, relaxed state of sedation. The ability to titrate N_2O is a significant advantage because it limits the amount of drug to that which is required by the patient. If titration is done properly, the patient does not receive any more of the drug than is necessary. Occasionally patients have had negative experiences with N_2O/O_2 sedation. In such cases the operator most likely did not titrate the amount of N_2O necessary to make the patient comfortable; instead, the patient received an inappropriate amount of drug, which usually causes oversedation. The concept of titration is the single most important skill to be learned in order to be a competent, safe administrator of any drug by any route.

XOX

I. Significance

A. It is extremely desirable to provide only the amount of a drug necessary for the procedure being performed. This allows for the expeditious elimination of the drug from the system, but more importantly, it creates a positive experience for the patient. With careful titration, vigilant monitoring of the patient, and updated equipment, negative experiences with N_2O/O_2 sedation should be rare.

B. Titration is very important when administering any drug. It minimizes the chances of a severe, possibly life-threatening, reaction should the patient be allergic to the drug. Fortunately, since the discovery of N_2O no allergic reaction to the drug has been reported.

C. Titration allows for biologic variability. No two humans are alike, and the same individual may give a very different response on a given day. Therefore habitually dispensing

10 mg Valium, 50 mg Demerol, or using 40% N_2O must be avoided because patient response cannot be guaranteed.

D. Sometimes idiosyncratic reactions may be encountered that are untoward and inexplicable (e.g., excitement after receiving a sedative drug). Titrating the drug would uncover such responses and minimize unexpected reactions immediately.

E. Titration can be applied to other drugs as well. For example, staggering local anesthetic injections over time allows for biotransformation tailored to the procedure and the patient's physiology. Titrating the dose of a drug is the considerate way to treat a patient individually.

II. *Adjusting Levels Appropriately*

A. Unique to N_2O is the ability to adjust levels of sedation quickly. Because of this important pharmacologic property, the onset of clinical effects is rapid. Signs and symptoms of sedation may be missed if close attention is not given.

B. Titration also allows for prolonged procedures to be accomplished effectively.

　　1. For example, when a potentially painful phase of treatment approaches, the nitrous gas may be increased. And conversely, as the intensity of the treatment subsides the nitrous gas can be decreased.

　　2. As the procedure nears completion, amounts of N_2O being delivered should be minimal. Because a minimum of 3 to 5 minutes of postoxygenation is required, it is appropriate to terminate the flow of N_2O and deliver 100% O_2 before completion of the procedure.

C. Remember that because of individual biovariability patients will require different levels of N_2O on different days and for different procedures.

　　1. The percentage of N_2O noted in a patient's chart from his/her last visit is irrelevant for the current appointment.

　　2. The most common mistake made with N_2O/O_2 sedation is to automatically deliver a preset percentage of N_2O to a patient. Remember, negative patient experiences from N_2O/O_2 sedation are most likely because the patient was oversedated as a result of operator error. Far too often patients blame any negative experience on the drug itself.

13

Technique for Nitrous Oxide/Oxygen Administration

It is extremely important to know the fundamentals of the technique for administering nitrous oxide/oxygen (N_2O/O_2). If you follow these basic principles, you can be assured that the experience will be positive for you and the patient. For decades these basic principles have not been followed, and too frequently negative patient experiences resulted. Concomitantly, operator frustration and lack of confidence occurred. It may take several positive experiences for a patient to become convinced that previous uncomfortable experiences with N_2O were caused not by nitrous oxide but rather by its administration. The technique is not difficult; observing patient response and being aware of the level of sedation are keys to success.

I. Fundamental Principles for Appropriate Administration

A. Be enthusiastic and confident that the experience will be positive. Your attitude will transfer to the patient.

B. Confidence is primarily preparation reflected in the individual who is informed and educated about nitrous oxide pharmacokinetics. Be knowledgeable about the limits of N_2O.

C. Recognize that a patient in your care represents the best opportunity you have to express genuine care and concern. Patients are more likely to refer others to you after a good experience.

D. Informed consent must be obtained for each patient before each N_2O/O_2 administration.

E. Practice titration. The amount of N_2O required by a patient on any given day or time varies. Do not adopt the fixed-dose philosophy; the amount of N_2O required on the previous visit means nothing for this appointment (see Chapter 12).

F. The procedure begins and ends with 100% pure O_2.

G. The patient should not be left alone. The effects of central nervous system (CNS) depression may be quick and/or subtle;

constant monitoring must be done by a professional trained in N_2O/O_2 sedation.

H. Accurate documentation of all procedures, reactions, complications, etc. must be maintained in the patient's file.

I. Because the final objective of the procedure is patient comfort, the patient should be placed in a comfortable position.

  1. To begin, depending on the discipline and the area of the body to be treated, the patient should be relaxed in a basic physiologic position.

  2. The upper torso should be slightly reclined and the legs slightly elevated. This can be easily accomplished with an adjustable chair. If a bed is used, prop the patient's head with pillows.

J. Inform the patient to ask for assistance at any time in the procedure if needed. The patient is the only person able to accurately state his/her feelings. You must honor the patient's trust by acknowledging each request.

K. If N_2O/O_2 is to be given at a subsequent appointment, advise the patient to avoid eating a big meal before that appointment. The presence of stomach contents does not precipitate vomiting; however, if vomiting occurs, emptying a full stomach will be embarrassing for the patient. The propensity for vomiting is higher in children than in adults.[1]

II. *Preoperative Unit Preparation*

A. Your N_2O/O_2 sedation armamentarium should include all equipment necessary to provide safe sedation experiences for the patient and a safe environment for the operator and all other exposed personnel.

  1. This equipment should be current, accurate, and include all available components for minimizing trace gas contamination.

  2. This will include an accurate flowmeter, scavenging masks, and a vacuum system able to eliminate gases at a rate of at least 45 L per minute.[2]

B. Ensure vacuum and ventilation exhaust are vented to the outside; make sure they are not near fresh-air intake vents.[2]

C. Assess the room/area ventilation.[2] The recirculating of room air is not recommended. A nonrecirculating ventilation system should be used to ensure that waste gases will not be circulated elsewhere within the building. If possible, create fresh air exchanges periodically. Opening a window to the outside is an easy way to provide fresh air; however, not all operatories have windows that can be opened. Use oscillating room fans near the floor to sweep waste gases out of the area and/or to the outside.

D. Confirm the absence of leaks at pressure connections on the unit. Bubbles will appear at leaking locations when a soap/water solution is used.

1. This procedure is recommended each time a cylinder is changed.

2. High-pressure lines should also be assessed periodically. The American Dental Association (ADA) expert panel recommends that this be done quarterly.[2]

3. Inspect the conducting tubing, reservoir bag, and their connections for leaks. These rubber products are subject to ultraviolet light degradation and should be visually inspected before each use. New silicone products appear to be more durable.

E. Connect disinfected conducting tubing with the disinfected reservoir bag if they are not already in place. Use recommended infection control measures; barriers may be used to cover units or sprayed/wiped with hospital-grade germicide. However, make sure the flowmeter can be easily read through the barrier.

F. Open the O_2 valve on the cylinder using the wrench (provided with the equipment) or knob (Figure 13-1). The pressure-gauge indicator (Figure 13-2) will rise and stop; this will alert you to the amount of O_2 in the tank. Turn on the N_2O/O_2 machine.

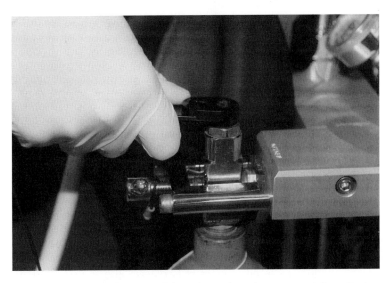

Figure 13-1 Open the O_2 tank by turning the valve on top of the cylinder.

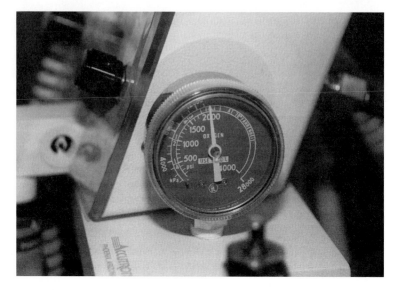

Figure 13-2 O_2 pressure gauge indicating cylinder contents.

1. If there is no O_2, the machine is nonfunctional until it becomes available.
2. Once O_2 is available to the system, the N_2O tank can then be opened in the same manner. The pressure-gauge indicator for the N_2O tank will read approximately 750 psi (Figure 13-3) unless the tank is nearly empty.
3. O_2 must be available at all times for the N_2O to flow. The operator must always be aware of the O_2 level in order to prevent unit shutdown intraoperatively.

G. Activate the portion of the scavenging system that involves placing the end of the conduction tubing into the evacuation or vacuum system (Figure 13-4).

1. Adjust the level of suction so that it does not pull the gas away from the patient or allow waste gas into the atmosphere.
2. If the suction level is even slightly above minimum, the N_2O/O_2 will be scavenged and thus not available to the patient. Keep the suction low.
3. Manufacturing companies are currently marketing monitoring devices that indicate the optimal evacuation level of 45 L per minute. One device is mounted close to the flowmeter; others may be found at the end of the conduction tubing before it is placed into the vacuum. To

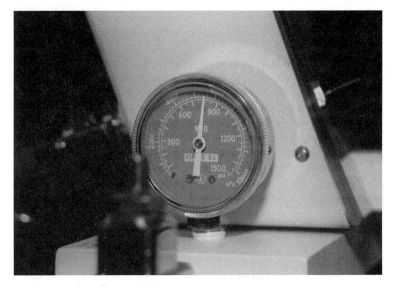

Figure 13-3   N₂O pressure gauge indicating cylinder contents.

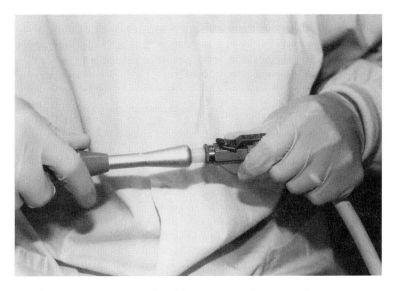

Figure 13-4   Engaging the delivery unit to the evacuation system.

date, these devices are not absolute, and improvement is needed to ensure reliable accuracy.

H. Using the O_2 flush button, partially inflate the reservoir bag to approximately two thirds full (Figure 13-5, *A*). Turn off the O_2 flush (Figure 13-5, *B*). The O_2 will continue to flow to the machine.

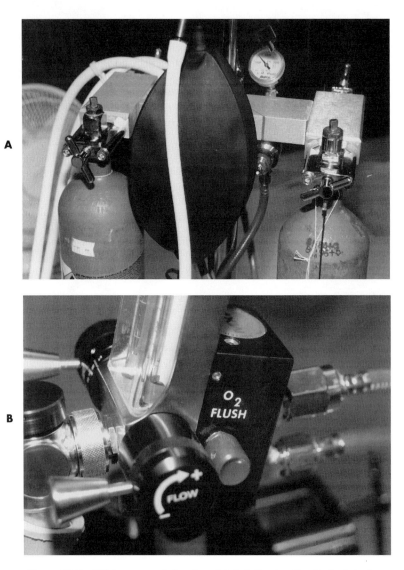

Figure 13-5   Fill the reservoir bag two thirds full using the O_2 flush button.

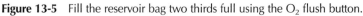

III. *Patient Participation*

A. Obtain the baseline vital signs of blood pressure (Figure 13-6, *A*), pulse (Figure 13-6, *B*), and respirations. Record these values on the sedation record or in the patient's chart.

B. Select the appropriate size and type of breathing apparatus for the patient. If using a scavenging nasal hood, find the size and/or scent most desirable to the patient. If using a full face mask, select the appropriate size and have the patient become familiar with it.

C. Adjust the O_2 flow to the system. According to the size, and physical/physiologic condition of the patient, estimate the total liters flow per minute (lpm).

    1. For an average-size adult, begin with 6 to 7 lpm (Figure 13-7). It is best to err with more flow than less flow initially to avoid a suffocating feeling. As the patient becomes relaxed, you may find that less flow is adequate.

    2. Begin with 4 to 5 lpm for most children.

    3. Set the machine to deliver the amount of 100% O_2 you have chosen. To ensure that there is flow, listen for the sound of O_2 moving into the breathing apparatus.

D. Secure the nasal hood or face mask and place it on the patient. Ask him/her to assist you in obtaining a snug but comfortable fit.

    1. Instruct the patient to adjust it at any time throughout the procedure. Allowing the patient this option gives him/her a sense of control.

    2. Adjust the conducting tubes behind the patient's head to ensure a snug fit (Figure 13-8). This will decrease the amount of air leaking from the mask.

        a. Take care not to tighten the apparatus so that patient movement is prohibited or pressure marks appear on his/her face.

        b. A piece of gauze may be folded over the patient's nose to minimize gas leakage should adjustment be inadequate, or the nasal hood may be trimmed to better fit the patient's anatomic features.

    3. Not only does an improper fit waste gas, but trace gas leakage contaminates the clinician's immediate environment (breathing zone).

E. Determine the appropriate amount of tidal volume needed for the patient. As the patient is breathing O_2, ask questions about the adequacy of the flow.

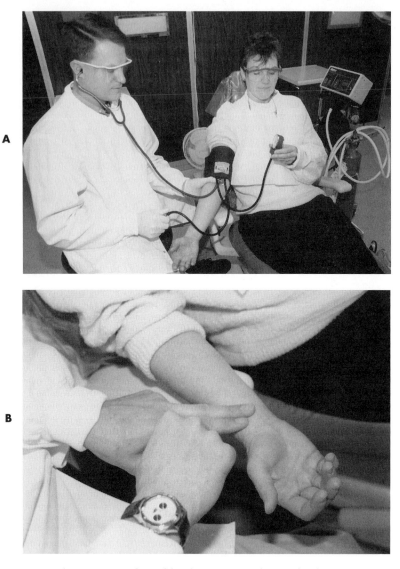

Figure 13-6 Obtain blood pressure reading and pulse rate.

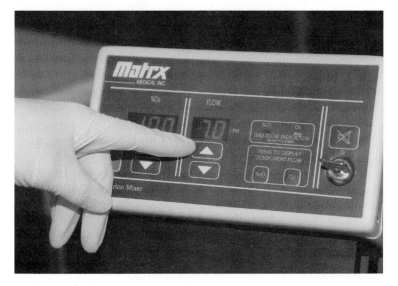

Figure 13-7 Establish the appropriate tidal volume for the patient.

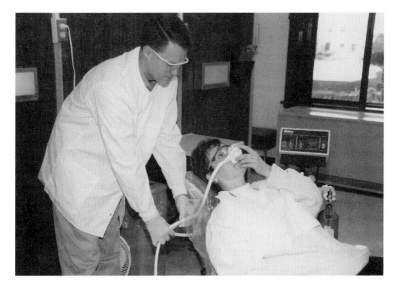

Figure 13-8 Secure the nasal hood to the patient.

1. Determine if the flow is sufficient to enable the patient to breathe comfortably. Also determine if the patient feels that there is too much gas flowing unnecessarily.
2. The reservoir bag is a good indicator for appropriate flow.[2]
   a. If the bag is bulging (Figure 13-9), decrease the lpm.
   b. If the bag continues to inflate like a balloon, it is possible that flow has been blocked somehow (Figure 13-10). Sometimes the bag may get caught between cylinders or the nonrebreathing valve may stick. Attend to this situation quickly.
   c. If the bag is collapsing, increase the lpm, check the seal around the patient's nose/face, and/or decrease the amount of vacuum to the unit.

F. It is important to instruct the patient to minimize talking during N_2O/O_2 sedation. Mouth breathing and talking will prevent the inhalation of gases into the patient's body, thereby reducing their effect and contaminating the immediate environment.

IV. Steps for Administration

A. Observe the reservoir bag periodically during the procedure for signs of patient respiration and assess the patient for comfort of gas flow; confirm the appropriate vacuum flow rate as well.[2] Depending on the type of machine and the preferred method of administration, there are two variations in the administration technique.
   1. If there are two controls on the machine that independently adjust the levels of each gas, the operator may choose to establish a constant O_2 flow level and add N_2O to the O_2 amount, or to establish the total lpm and adjust both gases by decreasing the O_2 and increasing the N_2O.
      a. The constant O_2 level technique would indicate an adjustment of O_2 to a level upon which N_2O would be added.
         i. For an average-size adult, 5 lpm may be an appropriate level. As N_2O is added, the total lpm will increase according to the amount of N_2O delivered. For example, the O_2 flow is set at 5 lpm, and 2 lpm N_2O is given; the total lpm is then 7.
         ii. The O_2 flow rate will remain constant. The total lpm will increase as N_2O is added.

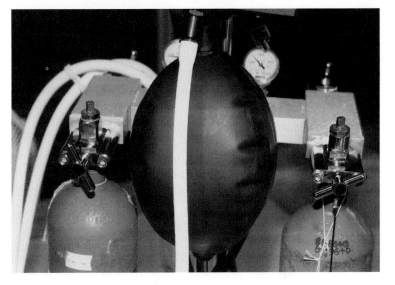

Figure 13-9   Reduce the tidal volume if the reservoir bag is bulging.

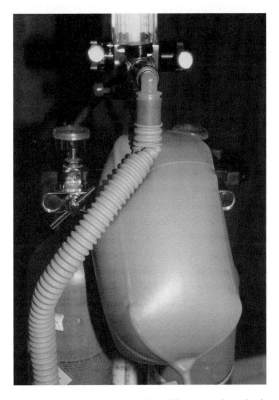

Figure 13-10   Be aware of potential problems, such as kinking hoses.

      iii. This technique allows for only one knob to be adjusted. Patients rarely complain of a suffocating feeling because large quantities of gas are delivered.

      iv. Because large quantities of gas are delivered some may leak around the nasal hood/face mask and contaminate the environment. In addition, the gas that is lost to the atmosphere is expensive.

  b. The other method of delivering N_2O and O_2 is done by decreasing the O_2 while increasing the N_2O.

      i. Following this technique will allow the total lpm to remain constant at the approximate level previously established.

      ii. Your machine may adjust the level of O_2 for you and deliver the total lpm that you establish. Once the total flow is determined, the machine will automatically decrease the amount of O_2 as you increase the amount of N_2O.

2. It is critical to remember that no matter which technique is being used, the lpm **does not** represent the percentage of N_2O being delivered. The actual percentage of N_2O is calculated by dividing the N_2O lpm by the total lpm.

  a. These figures have been calculated for you and are available in grid and table forms for your convenience. Examples of these forms can be found in Appendix B and may be photocopied, laminated, and attached to your machine or placed in your operatory.

  b. On machines that have the percent of O_2 displayed, it is necessary to subtract the number from 100 to obtain the percent of N_2O being delivered. For example: when 60% O_2 is displayed, 40% N_2O is being delivered.

B. Slow titration of N_2O is a must. Start with 10% N_2O or approximately 1 L and allow a minimum of 30 to 60 seconds for manifestation of clinical effects before adding additional N_2O. Instruct the patient to breathe through his/her nose, keeping the lips sealed.

1. During this time the operator will be questioning the patient about signs and symptoms. Advise the patient to refrain from excessive talking. As sedation deepens, note hypernasality of the voice resulting from the increased pressure of the gas on the tympanic membrane. Be wary of slurred speech, incoherence, nausea, or the inability

to verbally respond, as these signs indicate an inappropriate level of sedation.

2. Until the ideal sedation level is reached for that patient at that time, continue to add N_2O in increments of 5% or approximately ½ L with a 30- to 60-second minimum pause between increments.

C. Titrate to a level of sedation that is determined by patient comfort and relaxation.

1. There is no preset percentage for N_2O/O_2 sedation for a given patient or experience.

2. There is no preset lpm of N_2O/O_2 for a given patient or experience.

3. The percentage of N_2O given to a patient for a given experience will not reflect the amount necessary for any other experience. Individual biovariability will account for this variation in amount. Using a prescribed or previously administered amount may oversedate the patient and cause a negative experience unfairly blamed on the N_2O.

D. Intraoperative monitoring includes vigilant observation of the patient's responses and reactions in addition to observation of the reservoir bag.

1. The reservoir bag serves as a monitor of the patient's respirations. The bag will inflate and deflate slightly with the patient's inhalations and exhalations. Use this as a sign of conscious breathing.

2. Cumulative effects of N_2O may be seen as the duration of delivery increases. The level of sedation may deepen, resulting in uncomfortable symptoms for the patient.

3. Levels of sedation may fluctuate if the patient is allowed to maintain conversation and breathe through his/her mouth. This may produce a "roller coaster" effect, which can initiate nausea.

E. Perform procedures to be completed. The goal is to keep the patient relaxed and comfortable.

1. Adjust the level of N_2O as needed depending on the intensity of the procedures and the responses of the patient.

2. You may decrease the N_2O incrementally to a lesser amount for certain nonstimulating phases of treatment or completely if you are nearing completion of treatment. The patient may not realize your actions and incur a placebo effect.

F. When you terminate the N_2O flow, continue delivering 100% O_2 during final minutes of the procedure. This begins your required postoperative oxygenation period of 3 to 5 minutes (minimum). It is vital to pay close attention to this minimum time period (Figure 13-11).

1. It is unnecessary and inappropriate to use the O_2 flush button to remove the admixture of gases from the bag in order to provide 100% O_2, as this contaminates the environment with the N_2O. The technique of lifting the nasal hood off of the patient and purging the contents of the reservoir bag by squeezing it (Figure 13-12) also represents an inappropriate technique and is not recommended.[2]

2. To begin the postoxygenation period of 100% O_2, simply terminate the flow of N_2O and continue the flow of O_2.

3. If you administer O_2 for the required time during the final nonintensive phase of the procedure, the patient may be dismissed as soon as the procedure is completed rather than having to wait while you begin the postoxygenation period.

G. Assess the recovery of the patient. See Chapter 15 for specific details on recovery procedures.

1. If the patient senses any lethargy, dizziness, lightheadedness, or headache, continue 100% O_2 for additional minutes.

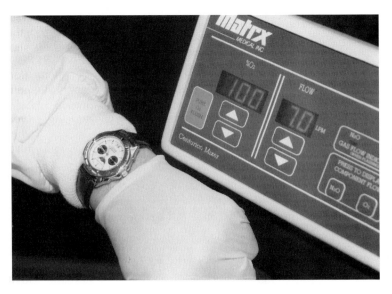

Figure 13-11 Postoperative oxygenation is mandatory for a minimum of 3 to 5 minutes.

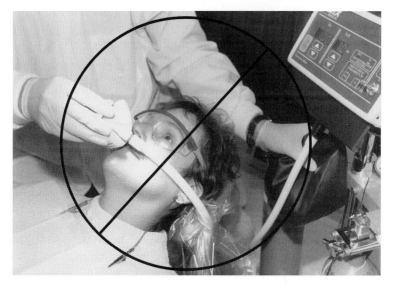

Figure 13-12 Do not purge the contents of the reservoir bag before postoxygenation; this contaminates the operator's breathing zone unnecessarily.

    2. When the patient feels normal, remove the breathing apparatus and allow the patient to breathe room air.

H. Obtain postoperative vital signs. Extend your appreciation of the patient's cooperation and trust. Reinforce the success of the appointment, then dismiss the patient.

V. *Postoperative Procedures*

A. It is important to record information regarding the sedation procedure in the patient's file just as you would document delivering local anesthesia or performing an operative procedure. Careful and thorough documentation is necessary for each patient. The following section provides details of record-keeping procedures.

B. For the N_2O line to bleed on portable units, O_2 must still be available. Remember to turn off the N_2O tank first. Use a wrench to close the valve; the pressure-gauge indicator should drop to zero. Close the valve on the O_2 tank and watch for the indicator to drop. Large tanks used with central supply units should be turned off at the end of the day. Turn off all master controls.

C. Perform all recommended disposal, disinfection, and sterilization procedures for the equipment. Consult the manufacturer's instructions for specific recommendations.

D. A condensed version of the administration technique can be found in Appendix B.

VI. *Prudent Record Keeping Procedures*

A. Importance
1. The primary purpose for keeping accurate and complete records in a healthcare setting is to provide a written history of patient/operator interactions. This runs the gamut—from the patient's health history, medications, and chief concerns to treatment options, completed procedures, recommendations, and much more.
2. This history will give an account for future reference to yourself or others so that the patient will receive continuity of care.
3. It is also a written record of chronologic events and experiences, making it a medicolegal document able to be used for you or against you in a court of law.

B. Fundamental principles of record keeping
1. A basic rule of thumb when making entries in a record is to write legibly so that others can read what is written.
2. Use a form of ink or marker (preferably black) that is permanent.
3. Make sure all services performed are recorded in a single location within the file in order to ensure a chronologic list.
4. Placing the name of the patient on each page in the file prevents lost information should a page become unattached.
5. If an error is made while recording information, draw two horizontal lines through the text and continue. Do not scribble through or use any type of correction material to cover what has been written. The information must still be legible even though it is erroneous. Otherwise, it may appear suspicious or altered.
6. The patient's file is a record of events occurring in chronologic order. Therefore it is important not to skip lines between entries. Spaces can be misconstrued as procedures unaccounted for between appointments.
7. It is recommended that the person making an entry in a patient's record sign or initial the entry. This will hold all

individuals accountable for the information, or lack thereof, that is written or unwritten.
C. Completing the N_2O/O_2 sedation record
　1. Specific information obtained during N_2O/O_2 sedation should be recorded in the patient's file. This information may be recorded as part of the appointment entry on the patient's service record or on a separate form. The following is a list of items to include in the patient's file for each experience.
　　a. Current date
　　b. Patient's name and age
　　c. Reason for N_2O/O_2 use (e.g., anxiety, hypersensitive gag reflex)
　　d. Notes from another health professional if consultation was necessary
　　e. The operative procedure being completed
　　f. Both preoperative and postoperative vital signs (blood pressure, pulse, and respiration)
　　g. Patient's tidal volume
　　h. Time N_2O flow began and ended
　　i. Peak percentage of N_2O administered
　　j. Amount of time (in minutes) postoxygenation was required for patient recovery
　　k. Any negative experiences or adverse conditions from the experience
　2. If a separate form is used, it must be permanently attached to the patient's file. A new form is to be used for each experience.
　3. An example of a N_2O/O_2 sedation record can be found in Appendix B. It may be photocopied for office use.

REFERENCES

1. Malamed SF: *Sedation: a guide to patient management,* ed 3, St Louis, 1995, Mosby.
2. American Dental Association Council on Scientific Affairs: Nitrous oxide in the dental office, *J Am Dent Assoc,* 128:364-365, 1997.

14

Signs and Symptoms of Nitrous Oxide/Oxygen Sedation

Individual biovariability accounts for different reactions to various amounts of nitrous oxide (N_2O). Some individuals will experience several symptoms; others only a few. Symptoms may be intense for some while insignificant for others. There will be instances when symptoms will be obvious; others will be subtle. Keeping a constant vigil is imperative when administering nitrous oxide/oxygen (N_2O/O_2) sedation because pleasant sensations may quickly become unpleasant. Your knowledge of the appropriate technique and associated physiologic/psychologic changes will increase your confidence with this procedure. Your ultimate goal is to increase patient comfort through relaxation.

I. Low N_2O Percentages/High O_2 Levels (Stage I)

A. Certain *physical/psychologic* effects may manifest in individuals when low percentages of N_2O are given accompanied by high O_2 levels.

1. The patient will express, overtly and/or inadvertently, an apparent sense of relaxation.
2. The patient will be happy, comfortable, and aware of his/her surroundings.
3. The patient will respond rationally and coherently to the operator's inquiry or directions. He/she will be able to maintain conversation; however, it is important to stress that the patient remain silent in order to receive the drug's effects.
4. If asked, the patient will acknowledge a reduced sense of fear/anxiety.
5. The individual's eyes may get a glazed or twinkling look, which is often accompanied by a big smile (Figure 14-1).

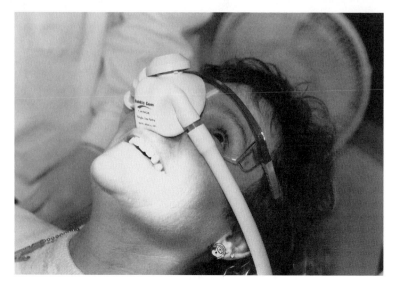

Figure 14-1   Stage I—Analgesia/Sedation.

6. If a local anesthetic injection is to be given for the procedure, the operator can ask the patient, "Would this be
a good time to give the injection?" The appropriately
sedated patient will acknowledge when this can occur
and will be very accepting of the procedure. We can
attest to the success of this technique as it has proven
quite reliable in our practices.

B. Several *physical/physiologic* effects may be present in varying degrees when low percentages of N_2O are given with
high levels of O_2.

1. A tingling may be felt in the fingers, toes, cheeks, lips,
tongue, head, or chest area. Some, all, or none of these
areas may be affected; therefore one should not pose
questions as to the presence of this symptom. Questions
should be goal-oriented, focusing on how the patient is
feeling rather than what the patient is feeling.

2. There may be noted heaviness in the patient's thighs
and/or legs. This sensation may be followed by a lighter,
floating feeling.

3. Because of the drug's effect on the tympanic membrane,
the patient's voice may resonate or carry a hypernasal
tone.

4. Patients may become warm, and their cheeks may flush as vasodilatation occurs.

II. *Increased N₂O Percentages/Moderate O₂ Levels (Stage II)*

A. As N_2O concentrations are increased, the *physical/psychologic* effects noted at lower levels may intensify or disappear. Some sensations will continue to be pleasant; however, changes may occur rapidly.

1. Relaxed states may develop into fits of uncontrolled laughing and giddiness. When this occurs, the patient will be primarily mouth-breathing, which could change the level of sedation. This may result in the roller coaster effect in which nausea can develop.

2. The patient may no longer feel he/she is in the same surroundings. A detachment or disassociation from the environment is possible.

3. The pleasant warmness felt in earlier states may intensify and become uncomfortable. The patient may express various signs of being too warm or even hot.

4. The patient may sense additional noises such as humming or vibrating sensations. This may simply be distracting or become bothersome.

5. Often patients will indicate lightweight or floating sensations. These may accompany the environmental detachment. They may feel an out-of-body experience.

B. The *physical/physiologic* effects of increasing N_2O concentrations become uncomfortable in some individuals. It is important to closely monitor the patient and be prepared to decrease N_2O concentrations immediately.

1. The patient may become very drowsy, which is not to be confused with being relaxed. He/she may actually want to sleep or appear to be in a dreamlike state. Patients can become sluggish with their motions. Words may be slurred or repeated; sentences may not make sense.

2. Patients may state they are dizzy and/or lightheaded. Nausea may be a symptom for some people.

3. As the Stage II—Excitement phase approaches, the patient may show signs of being agitated or physically uncomfortable. He/she may become restless and fidgety. At times patients even become combative and/or violent.

III. *High N$_2$O Percentages/Low O$_2$ Levels (Stage III)*

A. High percentages of N$_2$O are not recommended and, for most individuals, not necessary. Again, the *physical/psychologic* effects exhibited previously may be dramatically intensified or have now disappeared.

   1. The patient may actually be dreaming and/or hallucinating. Patients may attempt to respond to voices, people, visual effects, etc.

   2. Sexual fantasizing may occur with high N$_2$O percentages. The ramifications of this occurrence are discussed in Chapter 16.

B. High concentrations of N$_2$O can produce physical/physiologic effects that can be serious, if not life threatening.

   1. Nausea will occur more frequently with high N$_2$O percentages than at lower levels.

   2. Vomiting may occur at these levels, with a higher propensity for vomiting in children. Silent regurgitation can lead to aspiration of vomitus. This situation demands immediate advanced medical attention.

   3. The patient will most likely not respond to verbal commands. Words will be incoherent.

   4. The patient can fluctuate between consciousness and unconsciousness or actually become unconscious. All healthcare personnel must be able to respond to this type of emergency situation; however, close attention to the patient would prevent this from occurring.

15

Recovery from Nitrous Oxide/Oxygen Sedation

Recovery from nitrous oxide/oxygen (N_2O/O_2) sedation is an important part of the sedation experience. There are several aspects to complete recovery from the drug. The literature holds a plethora of references regarding psychologic and psychomotor effects that occur during N_2O/O_2 administration.[1-9] The extent of psychologic and psychomotor effects during N_2O/O_2 sedation will not be the same for any two individuals. One can also surmise from the literature that time for complete recovery from these effects cannot be reliably assessed.[1-9] Return to physiologic normalcy from N_2O/O_2 sedation appears to be readily apparent; however, the prudent practitioner will acknowledge the potential for individual biovariability regarding all aspects of recovery and will act with common sense regarding patient dismissal from the clinical setting.

I. Principles of Recovery

A. Generally, emergence (recovery) is a mirror image of induction.[10] This mirror image includes the patient returning to his/her original emotional state as well as recovering from the pharmacologic action of the drug. N_2O evokes a rapid onset of clinical activity and thus a correlated rapid emergence from the sedation endpoint. Therefore providing a calm, tranquil preoperative environment will facilitate the sedative experience from beginning to end.

B. Physiologically, recovery occurs the same way for any individual. N_2O, as mentioned earlier, is principally exhaled unchanged from the lungs. Again, the potential exists for postoperative symptoms of lethargy, headache, and nausea to occur. While opinions vary among researchers as to whether these symptoms are caused by diffusion hypoxia, we believe that postoxygenation is required. Postoxygenation remains an extremely important concept of recovery. Postoperatively,

100% O_2 must be administered for a minimum of 3 to 5 minutes. Depending on individual biovariability, this post-oxygenation period may be extended until both patient and operator are satisfied that adequate recovery has been achieved.

II. Psychologic and Psychomotor Effects

A. Several studies have been completed by reputable professionals investigating the effects of N_2O on psychomotor ability, memory, mood, and cognition.[1-9] Many tests have been commonly used to assess these functions: visual analogue scales have been used to assess mood; psychomotor impairment has been assessed using digit-symbol substitution tests, paper/pencil tests, eye/hand coordination tests, automobile driving simulation, etc.; questionnaires have been used to ascertain degrees of euphoria, concentration, and attention. Results of these tests vary; however, experts agree that mental and psychomotor impairment does occur with N_2O, as it does with almost every other drug.

B. Psychologic and psychomotor impairment during N_2O/O_2 administration has been well established. We need to be assured to the greatest extent possible that patients are adequately recovered from sedation so they do not harm themselves or others upon dismissal from our offices. To date there are no references to cases in which patients who were dismissed after N_2O/O_2 sedation harmed or injured themselves or others because of incomplete recovery from the drug.

III. Technique for Assessing Adequate Recovery

A. It is important to remember that not all patients recover to the extent that they may be dismissed without an escort. Depending on the circumstances of the situation, an educated practitioner must make this decision based on knowledge of the drug effects and the patient.

B. The patient's response to questioning will be subjective but in most cases valid.

1. After the required postoxygenation period of 3 to 5 minutes minimum, you should begin questioning the patient about how he/she feels. The patient should indi-

cate that he/she is feeling relaxed but not drowsy, comfortable, etc.

2. If there is any indication that there is a deviation from normal feelings, or if negative responses are given, assume that recovery is not complete and additional postoxygenation time is required. All responses should be positive and should indicate normal feelings.

C. Postoperative vital signs are an objective measure of recovery.

1. Generally, blood pressure values within 10 mm Hg (both systolic and diastolic) from preoperative readings are considered to be within an accepted comparable range.

2. Likewise, a postoperative pulse rate within 10 beats and a respiration rate within 5 beats are acceptable parameters for comparison.

3. As mentioned earlier, a pulse oximeter can be used for obtaining and recording this information. This machine produces a paper printout that can be attached to the patient's record for documentation purposes.

D. Psychomotor recovery from inhalation sedation has been addressed in the literature.

1. Early studies[11-13] recommended preoperative and postoperative drawing tests to determine visual-motor coordination and recovery. In the studies, recovery was complete within 3 to 5 minutes after termination of the N_2O.[11-13]

2. Jastak and Orendurff[14] investigated psychomotor recovery by using a driving simulation test. Participants were evaluated for errors in steering, braking, signaling, and speeding. All postsedation figures correlated with presedation values, thereby concluding that patients could safely operate a motor vehicle after N_2O/O_2 sedation.[14] The study has been the foundation for practitioners dismissing patients without an escort.

3. There is a simple hand/eye coordination exercise that can be done in the office to assess psychomotor recovery. Have the patient extend his/her arm out to the side; then give instructions to place his/her little finger on the tip of his/her nose. The exercise may be done with either/both hands. Accuracy is subjective; however, if this simple skill cannot be completed, it may be necessary to reevaluate adequate recovery.

E. Responsibility lies in the hands of the operator to make an educated decision as to the complete recovery of the patient before his/her dismissal.

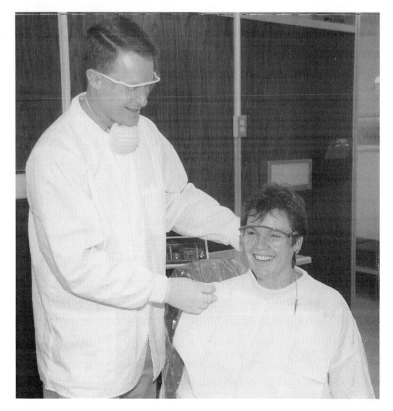

REFERENCES

1. Cheam EW et al: The effect of nitrous oxide on the performance of psychomotor tests: a dose-response study, *Anaesthesia* 50:764-768, 1995.

2. Fagan D et al: A dose-response study of the effects of inhaled nitrous oxide on psychological performance and mood, *Psychopharmacology* 116:333-338, 1994.

3. Dohrn CS et al: Subjective and psychomotor effects of nitrous oxide in healthy volunteers, *Behav Pharmacol* 3:19-30, 1992.

4. Armstrong PJ et al: Effects of nitrous oxide on psychological performance: a dose-response study using inhalation of concentrations up to 15%, *Psychopharmacology* 117:486-490, 1995.

5. Zacny JP et al: Time course of effects of brief inhalations of nitrous oxide in normal volunteers, *Addiction* 89:831-839, 1994.

6. Zacny JP et al: The subjective, behavioral and cognitive effects of subanesthetic concentrations of isoflurane and nitrous oxide in healthy volunteers, *Psychopharmacology* 114:409-416, 1994.

7. Yajnik S et al: Effects of marijuana history on the subjective, psychomotor, and reinforcing effects of nitrous oxide in humans, *Drug Alcohol Depend* 36:227-236, 1994.

8. Tiplady R, Sinclair WA, Morrison LM: Effects of nitrous oxide on psychological performance, *Psychopharmacol Bull* 28:207-211, 1992.

9. Ramsay JS et al: Paradoxical effects of nitrous oxide on human memory, *Psychopharmacology* 106:370-374, 1992.

10. Eger EI II: Uptake and distribution. In Miller RD, editor: *Anesthesia,* vol 1, ed 4, New York, 1994, Churchill Livingstone.

11. Newman MG, Trieger N, Miller JC: Measuring recovery from anesthesia: a simple test, *Anesth Anal* 48:136-140, 1969.

12. Trieger N, Newman MG, Miller JC: An objective measure of recovery, *Anesth Prog* 16:4-7, 1969.

13. Trieger N et al: Nitrous oxide: a study of physiological and psychomotor effects, *J Am Dent Assoc* 82:142-150, 1971.

14. Jastak JT, Orendurff D: Recovery from nitrous sedation, *Anesth Prog* 22:113-116, 1975.

16

Nitrous Oxide Abuse Issues

Nitrous oxide (N$_2$O) has been used for recreational purposes since its discovery in the late eighteenth century. Sir Humphrey Davy and Dr. Gardner Colton traveled the world proclaiming the exhilarating effects of inhaling N$_2$O in those early days. Inhaling the gas was popular at social gatherings during that time and is still done at parties today. N$_2$O abuse is not as significant as abuse of other drugs but is nonetheless an issue about which healthcare professionals should be aware. When chronically abused, N$_2$O can have serious health ramifications. N$_2$O should be given the same respect that is given to all drugs.

I. Inhalant Abuse

A. All drugs that produce euphoria have the potential to be abused, whether they are injected, swallowed, or inhaled.

B. Inhaling chemicals found in a variety of household products is a method of achieving a quick, exhilarating high. It is particularly unfortunate that this type of inhalant abuse appears to be most common among children and adolescents. Studies in the 1980s indicated that 18.6% of United States high school seniors had practiced inhaling chemicals at least once; specific states claimed even higher incidence figures and younger users.[1] A 1993 report from the National Institute on Drug Abuse (NIDA) indicates approximately 17% of U.S. adolescents say they have sniffed inhalants.[2] For youth and others who may be disadvantaged financially, inhalants present a way of "getting high" that is cheap and easily attained.[1]

C. These younger users claim a variety of favorite inhalant products. Euphoria-producing chemicals, found in commonly used products, are readily available.

1. Examples of products that are inhaled include fuels such as gasoline, butane, and propane; solvents; paint and

paint thinner; rubber cement; airplane glue; hair spray; shoe polish; nail polish remover; deodorants; lubricating cooking sprays; insect repellent; and typewriter correction fluid.

2. Typewriter correction fluid is one of the favored inhalants. It contains the chemical 1,1,1-trichloroethane or trichloroethylene. Through 1988, abuse of this substance was responsible for 27 reported fatalities. A leading manufacturer incorporated mustard oil into its product to discourage abuse.[1] Health risks from inhaling this product include liver damage, cranial neuropathy, and cardiac toxicity.[1]

D. Many inhalants are central nervous system (CNS) depressants that produce sensations similar to the effects of sedation and anesthesia. However, abusers are looking for the exhilarating, euphoric, visually stimulating effects. Effects are produced in less than 1 minute and are usually not long lasting. Some experienced users claim to feel effects for up to 45 minutes and can therefore time their experiences to prolong their exuberance for hours.[1] Disorientation can occur; nausea and vomiting have been reported, as well as sneezing, coughing, and salivation.[3]

E. Obviously, these products are sold legally and are relatively inexpensive. They are found at home and in the garage. They are purchased in grocery, hardware, and drug stores. They can be packaged in small containers that are easily hidden. Most often, purchase of such products would pose no suspicion. However, in some areas, local sale restrictions may apply if there is a known or suspected abuse problem.

F. Other risk groups for abuse of these inhalants include those who may be occupationally exposed to the products. Those at risk may be janitors, painters, dry cleaning personnel, automobile repair workers, or hairstylists.[1]

G. Amyl nitrite and butyl nitrite ("poppers") are muscle relaxants inhaled primarily to intensify and prolong sexual experiences. Marketed as room deodorizers, these products may produce symptoms such as headaches, blurred vision, and cardiac arrhythmia.[1]

H. N_2O falls into the inhalant classification as well. It has similar pharmacokinetic properties to those products listed above. It is relatively inexpensive, readily accessible, legal to purchase, and produces a rapid, euphoric high. Users recommend its use to others claiming that it produces feelings of floating or flying; vivid, visual, colorful images; and loss of all inhibitions, making the user feel invincible. Of course the negative side effects like fatigue, fainting, nausea, and cardiac arrest are rarely mentioned.

II. N_2O *Abuse*

A. N_2O users tend to be somewhat older than those inhaling solvents and fuels, etc. As when it was first introduced, N_2O is popular today at college social activities such as parties and concerts and may be advertised in college papers or flyers. N_2O etiquette can be found in high-society magazines; reference to its use at elite parties can be found in novels. Now instructions for its use can be found even on the Internet.

B. Health professionals who have ready access to the gas are noted recreational users. In general, health professionals have access to many drugs, and abuse is often not limited to one drug. Anesthesiologists and those in training, students in psychiatric and maxillofacial programs, physicians, and dentists are groups cited in the literature as being substance abusers.[4,5] In a 1977 anonymous survey of medical and dental students 20% admitted to using N_2O socially.[6]

C. N_2O is considerably easy to obtain for recreational use and is found in several forms.

1. Because it is commonly found compressed in cylinders and used for medical/dental purposes, it is easy to locate in hospitals, clinics, dental offices, etc.

   a. Several agencies have reported stolen cylinders from such places. If an individual is employed in such a setting, he/she may be able to use the gas on site rather than taking the risk of stealing the cylinder.

   b. Distribution centers where cylinders of N_2O are filled and distributed to various sites report occasional robbery attempts. Large cylinders previously stored outside of buildings have been moved indoors for security.

2. N_2O is also used in the auto racing industry; it supports combustion and is used as an engine-boosting agent. However, nitrous oxide used for this purpose is often mixed with sulfur dioxide. Inhaling this noxious mixture is likely to render a person ill with vomiting, headache, and diarrhea.

3. Messina and Wynne,[7] researching homemade N_2O, produced the gas according to instructions widely distributed in "head shops" and claim that the process was easy and inexpensive. They also report that significant concentrations of nitrogen dioxide and nitric oxide are produced

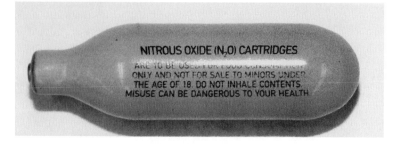

NITROUS OXIDE (N₂O) CARTRIDGES
ARE TO BE USED FOR FOOD CONSUMPTION
ONLY AND NOT FOR SALE TO MINORS UNDER
THE AGE OF 18. DO NOT INHALE CONTENTS.
MISUSE CAN BE DANGEROUS TO YOUR HEALTH

Figure 16-1 Whipping cream charger "whippet."

with this method. These substances are toxic and can cause transient pulmonary toxicity and tissue damage.

4. N_2O is approved by the Food and Drug Administration (FDA) as a food ingredient because the dairy industry uses it as a whipping cream propellant. The gas expands into the cream causing it to whip into a foam. When used for these legitimate purposes, N_2O is found in 3-inch long containers called *whippets* (Figure 16-1). These containers hold approximately 4 to 5 L of N_2O. These products are also misused for recreational purposes.

   a. In addition to the whippet charger, a "cracker" and a balloon must be purchased (Figure 16-2). A balloon is attached to one end while the charger is placed between the two halves of the cracker. A pointed extension inside the cracker pierces the diaphragm on the charger as the two halves are screwed together. The gas is expelled out of the charger and fills the balloon.

5. Similarly, approximately 3 L of N_2O is found in aerosol cans of whipping cream. It is the N_2O that whips the cream coming out of the can. Figure 16-3 illustrates N_2O listed as a propellant.

   a. This event becomes a game as users try to "hit" off of a can in a grocery store without buying the product. This "grocery store high" was reported in the psychiatric literature in 1978.[8] Restaurants have reported the necessity for locking the supply of whipping cream cans to prevent servers from sampling the N_2O while on the job.

   b. To prohibit inhaling N_2O from the aerosol can without purchasing it, manufacturers have indicated they will wrap the entire can in tamper-resistant plastic.

   c. N_2O can also be found in chargers that are similar in size to a seltzer bottle. Again, the legitimate use is for

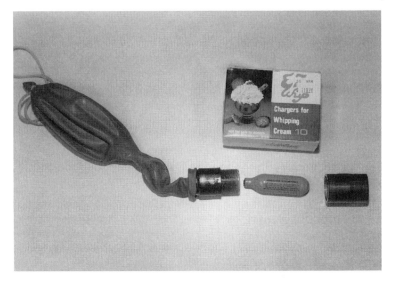

Figure 16-2 Whippet assembly for recreational misuse.

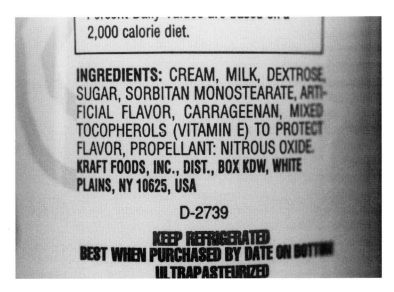

... Percent Daily Values are based on a
2,000 calorie diet.

INGREDIENTS: CREAM, MILK, DEXTROSE, SUGAR, SORBITAN MONOSTEARATE, ARTIFICIAL FLAVOR, CARRAGEENAN, MIXED TOCOPHEROLS (VITAMIN E) TO PROTECT FLAVOR, PROPELLANT: NITROUS OXIDE. KRAFT FOODS, INC., DIST., BOX KDW, WHITE PLAINS, NY 10625, USA

D-2739

KEEP REFRIGERATED
BEST WHEN PURCHASED BY DATE ON BOTTOM
ULTRAPASTEURIZED

Figure 16-3 Aerosol whipping cream can ingredient list; note the propellant listed is N_2O.

creating whipped cream; however, those misusing it inhale the contents directly from the bottle or dispel it into balloons.[9]

D. Because of the pharmacokinetics of the drug, N_2O is rarely detected in routine urine tests.[10] Therefore users may substitute N_2O for other more detectable drugs, especially when driving. However, there have been reports of youth involved in fatal car accidents when under the influence of the N_2O.[9]

✕✕✕

III. Health Hazards Associated with Chronic Exposure to N_2O

A. N_2O has been shown to affect vitamin B_{12} metabolism. It oxidizes the cobalt ion in the vitamin B_{12} cofactor, rendering the enzyme methionine synthase inactive in folate metabolic pathways. Methionine synthase plays a vital role in the production of deoxyribonucleic acid (DNA). Megaloblastic hematopoiesis and leukopenia result after prolonged exposure to nitrous oxide.[11]

1. For the surgical or ambulatory patient undergoing N_2O/O_2 sedation, the effects of inactivated methionine synthase are temporary and insignificant for the healthy individual. There appears to be a greater risk for pregnant women, those with impaired wound healing capabilities, and for those with existing vitamin B_{12} deficiencies.[11]

2. Studies on laboratory animals have shown that enzyme inactivation occurs rapidly during N_2O overexposure and that recovery is slow.[11,12] Animal studies have also shown evidence of fetal toxicity resulting in skeletal abnormalities and miscarriages after significant exposure to N_2O in terms of concentration and time.[11]

3. Several studies with humans revealed significant hematopoietic changes as well; the earliest report was cited in 1956.[13-15] Research has confirmed this consequence over the years. An excellent reference list to this subject can be found in Eger's text, *Nitrous Oxide, N_2O*.[16]

4. Individuals who are chronically exposed to N_2O through its recreational use or occupational use in unscavenged areas may be at risk for hematopoietic changes and other sequelae. Chapter 17 provides further details on the biohazard and scavenging issues associated with trace gas contamination.

5. Those persons who are vitamin B_{12} deficient may be affected as well; these persons may not be aware of the

deficiency until the N_2O exposure produces neurologic changes.[17]

    a. Vitamin B_{12} is found in foods that are high in fat. Because Americans are becoming increasingly fat-conscious, many persons may not consume an adequate amount of vitamin B_{12}.

    b. It has been suggested that a vitamin B_{12} supplement be taken by women exposed to N_2O as a method for reducing fetotoxic effects.[17] The possibility of biochemical protection exists for other compromised individuals as well. N_2O researchers agree that this is an area in need of continued study.

B. Neurologic side effects have been associated with chronic use of N_2O. Several reports in the literature cite peripheral neuropathy in individuals who indicate habitual use of N_2O.[18]

    1. Neurologic symptoms have been reported primarily by individuals who have admitted using N_2O recreationally; however, in some cases, affected individuals were exposed to significant amounts of unscavenged N_2O in hospitals or during dental surgery.[19] Symptoms relating to peripheral neuropathy are evidenced by tingling and numbness in the extremities, weakness and incoordination, lack of strength and dexterity in the hands, slowed gait, and positive Lhermitte's sign (electric shock feeling upon flexion of the neck).[20-22]

    2. Often the neuropathic symptoms are not immediate; they may appear several months into the overexposure period.[19] Generally, neurologic function slowly returns to normal after termination of overexposure to the gas. This return is gradual and in some cases may not be complete.[19]

    3. The cases of overexposure reported in the literature are primarily dentists or other health professionals who deliver N_2O to patients without proper scavenging equipment.[23] Other cases are young adults recreationally inhaling N_2O from whipping cream chargers.[20,23] Most of the overexposure incidents reported were periods of 1 to 2 hours per day, at least three times a week, and for periods of several months to years.[18,23] In some cases individuals reported falling asleep and incurring up to 4 hours of exposure; one individual admitted self-administration of 2 to 4 hours per day while another admitted 6 to 7 hours per day.[23]

C. Frostbite has been cited as a consequence of recreational exposure to N_2O. One case involved an anesthesiologist complaining of frostbitten hands and palms during employment. More significant are reports of individuals sniffing N_2O straight from the cylinder, causing their mouths, lips, and cheeks to freeze to the extent that tissue necrosed to a fourth-degree burn.[24] In one instance an individual became so disoriented from inhaling the gas that he was unaware that his cheek was in contact with the gas and cylinder for a prolonged period of time.[24]

D. There have been reports of pneumothorax or pneumomediastinum resulting from the pressure released from a whippet charger. In one instance, actual rupture of alveolar walls occurred, causing interstitial emphysema.[25]

E. Several reports of asphyxial death from N_2O are stated in the literature.[26-29] All victims were using N_2O recreationally. Several victims have been healthcare workers, others worked in restaurants, while some were users outside of the work place.

   1. The reported deaths of healthcare workers usually involve cylinder apparatus with face masks. Details surrounding the instances reveal victims being found near tanks in healthcare settings.

   2. Other reports describe victims being discovered with plastic bags over their heads and belts or similar devices around their necks to keep the bags closed. In these situations chargers are frequently used and are discharged inside the plastic bag.

      a. Wagner et al[10] recreated the scenario of discharging of a whipping cream charger inside a plastic bag. Within 10 seconds of discharging, the 21% O_2 concentration found in ambient air inside the bag had dropped to 13% and the N_2O concentration escalated to 59%. Within 1 minute the O_2 concentration had fallen to 10%.

      b. Unconsciousness occurs either from the hypoxia or the drug concentration, and death results when available O_2 is depleted to a level that does not support life.[10] Death by this means sometimes may be sought intentionally and other times may be accidental.

   3. In one case N_2O was implicated as the cause for an autoerotic asphyxial death. The victim had created a method of delivering N_2O through an outdated and modified anesthetic machine, and sexual material describing bondage and other autoerotic methods were found at the scene.[30]

IV. *Sexual Phenomena Associated with N_2O*

A. Euphoric effects have been associated with N_2O since it was first introduced. Some reports in the literature have indicated that hallucinations, visualizations, and auditory illusions have resulted from N_2O abuse.[31] There have also been situations in which aberrations of a sexual nature have been reported.[32]

   1. Allegations of sexual impropriety have been made against health professionals after patients were sedated with N_2O/O_2. These complaints were taken to court for prosecution, but in the majority of cases the charges were dismissed. However, licensure was subject to the discretion of the state's licensing board.

   2. Specific cases reported have been primarily against male practitioners by female patients. The cases report claims such as the patient falling asleep and being frightened by a visualization, pressure sensations in the genital region, becoming sexually stimulated, feeling naked, dreaming, and fantasizing.[32]

   3. Jastak and Malamed[32] report that in all of those instances concentrations of N_2O higher than 50% were used. They also indicate that no other personnel accompanied the dentist during the sedation experience.[32] They recommend that a third party be present at all times and that N_2O concentrations greater than 50% be avoided.[32]

   4. Lambert[33] suggests that hypnosis is potentiated by nitrous oxide. He suggests that a person may experience a hypnotic state spontaneously or by the suggestive language of the professional while N_2O is being administered. Lambert[33] recommends that the practitioner regard his/her statements in a professional manner without lending comments that could be misinterpreted. He recommends suggesting visual imagery such as a beach scene in order to avoid the patient's own imaging.

B. Obviously, the allegation of sexual impropriety can create uncomfortable situations. Use common sense when using N_2O; do not place yourself in potentially incriminating situations. Practice with a third party in the vicinity who is educated on the effects of N_2O. Titrate to the appropriate endpoint of sedation in order to avoid high concentrations of N_2O and oversedation symptoms.

V. *Addictive Nature of N_2O*

A. Compared with other drugs, nitrous oxide abuse is low.[9] It is not listed among the most commonly abused drugs. This drug has been used for 150 years without mention of significant abuse and addiction problems.

B. Evidence exists that suggests N_2O is involved with the endogenous opioid system directly at a receptor site and/or indirectly by activating opioid neurotransmitters.

　　1. Also indicated is the fact that N_2O may be considered a partial opioid agonist, making it less addictive than a full agonist such as morphine.[34]

　　2. Autotolerance may be an issue with N_2O, indicating that the body rapidly becomes tolerant to its effects.[10]

C. Compared with other drugs, N_2O abuse does not exist as a public health concern. Alcohol, nicotine, and cannabis have been cited as the most commonly used nonmedical drugs.[35] However, it is still important to be aware of its recreational use among youth and health professionals in particular.

VI. *Legislation/Regulation Issues*

A. Currently there are few regulations governing the sale or purchase of N_2O. Distributors are ethically obligated to confirm that their customers are purchasing the drug for appropriate use; however, there are no control measures to ensure that this is happening.

B. Warning labels can be found on cylinders, whippets, and whipping cream containers containing N_2O. The labels recommend that users be familiar with the administration and properties of the drug and that misuse could be harmful.

C. The Compressed Gas Association Foundation, the Compressed Gas Association (CGA), and the National Welding Supply Association (NWSA) have been active in informing the public about the concern of N_2O misuse. The Nitrous Oxide Abuse Task Force was established in 1994 by the CGA and NWSA. They created the Sales and Security Guidelines for the Safe Use/Handling of Nitrous Oxide.[36] The guidelines provide suggestions and information to producers, repackagers, distributors, carriers, and legitimate users of the gas. See Appendix A for references to this information. Fifty-nine associations were targeted by the task force to receive these guidelines. They range from healthcare and restaurants to auto racing, law enforcement, and trucking.

D. In addition to these guidelines, the CGA and NWSA are working with other organizations to tighten distribution policies and develop strong codes of ethics for voluntary implementation. They also provide assistance to those working with law enforcement individuals dealing with N_2O misuse issues.

E. Legislatively, these organizations have been instrumental in assisting the development of model state legislation that would discourage illicit N_2O use and make violations punishable by law. Several states have been on the forefront of this issue and have already been successful in enacting legal regulations. States to be commended for their involvement in this subject are Maryland, West Virginia, Illinois, California, and Georgia.

REFERENCES

1. Schwartz RJ: When to suspect inhalant abuse, *Patient Care* 30:39-64, 1989.
2. National Institute on Drug Abuse Website: www.nida.nih.gov.
3. McHugh MJ: The abuse of volatile substances, *Ped Clin North Am* 34:333-340, 1987.
4. Gillman MA: Nitrous oxide abuse in perspective, *Clin Neuropharmacol* 15: 297-306, 1992.
5. From RP: Substance dependence and abuse by anesthesia care providers. In Rogers M et al, editors: *Principles and practice of anesthesiology,* St Louis, 1993, Mosby.
6. Rosenberg H, Orkin FK, Springstead J: Abuse of nitrous oxide, *Anesth Analg* 58:104-106, 1979.
7. Messina FV, Wynne JW: Homemade nitrous oxide: no laughing matter, *Ann Int Med* 96:333-334, 1982.
8. Block SH: The grocery store high, *Am J Psychiatry* 135:126-127, 1978.
9. Murray MJ, Murray WJ: Nitrous oxide availability, *J Clin Pharm* 20:202-205, 1980.
10. Wagner SA et al: Asphyxial deaths from the recreational use of nitrous oxide, *J Forensic Sci* 37:1008-1015, 1992.
11. Nunn JF, Chanarin I: Nitrous oxide inactivates methionine synthetase. In Eger EI II: *Nitrous oxide N_2O,* New York, 1985, Elsevier Science Publishing.
12. Londo H, Osborne ML: Nitrous oxide has multiple deleterious effects on cobalamin metabolism and causes decreases in activities of mammalian cobalamin dependent enzymes, *J Clin Invest* 67:1270-1283, 1981.
13. Lassen JC et al: Treatment of tetanus: severe bone marrow depression after prolonged nitrous-oxide anaesthesia, *Lancet* 1:527-530, 1956.
14. Amess JA et al: Megaloblastic haemopoiesis in patients receiving nitrous oxide, *Lancet* 2:339-340, 1978.
15. Skacel PO et al: Studies on the haemopoietic toxicity of nitrous oxide in man, *Br J Haematol* 53:189-200, 1983.
16. Eger EI II: *Nitrous Oxide,* N_2O, New York, 1985, Elsevier Science Publishing.
17. Ostreicher JS: Vitamin B_{12} supplements as protection against nitrous oxide inhalation, *New York State Dent J* 60:47-49, 1994.
18. Kunkel DB: The toxic emergency, *Emerg Med* 19:79-84, 1987.
19. Layzer RB: Myeloneuropathy after prolonged exposure to nitrous oxide, *Lancet* 2:1227-1230, 1978.

20. Sahenk Z et al: Polyneuropathy from inhalation of N_2O cartridges through a whipped-cream dispenser, *Neurology* 28:485-487, 1978.

21. Layzer RB, Fishman RA, Schafer JA: Neuropathy following abuse of nitrous oxide, *Neurology* 28:504-506, 1978.

22. Paulson GW: "Recreational" misuse of nitrous oxide, *J Am Dent Assoc* 98:410-411, 1979.

23. Gutmann L, Johnsen D: Nitrous oxide-induced myeloneuropathy: report of cases, *J Am Dent Assoc* 103:239-241, 1981.

24. Hwang JC, Himel HN, Edlich RF: Frostbite of the face after recreational misuse of nitrous oxide, *Burns* 22:152-153, 1996.

25. LiPuma JP, Wellman J, Stern HP: Nitrous oxide abuse: a new cause for pneumomediastinum, *Radiology* 145:602, 1982.

26. Suruda AJ, McGlothlin JD: Fatal abuse of nitrous oxide in the workplace, *J Occup Med* 32:682-684, 1990.

27. Garriott J, Petty CS: Death from inhalant abuse: toxicological and pathological evaluation of 34 cases, *Clin Toxicology* 16:305-315, 1980.

28. Chadly A, Marc B, Barres D: Suicide by nitrous oxide poisoning, *Am J For Med Path* 10:330-331, 1989.

29. Winek CL, Wahba WW, Rozin L: Accidental death by nitrous oxide inhalation, *Forensic Sci Int* 73:139-141, 1995.

30. Leadbeatter S: Dental anesthetic death: an unusual autoerotic episode, *Am J For Med Path* 9:60-63, 1988.

31. Steinberg H: Abnormal behavior induced by nitrous oxide, *Br J Psychol* 47:183-194, 1956.

32. Jastak, JT, Malamed SF: Nitrous oxide sedation and sexual phenomena, *J Am Dent Assoc* 101:38-40, 1980.

33. Lambert C: Sexual phenomena hypnosis and nitrous oxide sedation, *J Am Dent Assoc* 101:990-991, 1982.

34. Gillman MA: Nitrous oxide, an opioid addictive agent, *Am J Med* 81:97-102, 1986.

35. Kreek MJ: Multiple drug abuse patterns and medical consequences. In Meltzer HY, editor: *Psychopharmacology: the third generation of progress,* New York, 1987, Raven Press.

36. Compressed Gas Association Code-201: *Nitrous oxide sales and security recommended guidelines,* Arlington, Va, 1995, Compressed Gas Association.

SUGGESTED READINGS

Dohrn CS et al: Reinforcing effects of extended inhalation of nitrous oxide in humans, *Drug Alcohol Depend* 31:265-280, 1993.

Dzoljic M et al: Behavioral and electrophysiological aspects of nitrous oxide dependence, *Brain Res Bull* 33:25-31, 1994.

Pollard TG: Relative addiction potential of major centrally-active drugs and drug classes—inhalants and anesthetics, *Advances in Alcohol and Substance Abuse* 9:149-165, 1990.

17

Potential Biohazards for Health Personnel Associated with Chronic Exposure to Nitrous Oxide

Nitrous oxide/oxygen (N_2O/O_2) sedation has already been discussed as being a safe procedure that will not pose health risks for a patient. However, chronic exposure for health professionals has been an issue of debate and concern for several years. This chapter provides current and accurate information to clarify this sometimes misunderstood and emotional issue.

I. History of Controversial Literature

A. In 1967 a Russian scientist named Vaisman[1] reported that both male and female anesthesiologists in this country experienced reproductive problems at a significantly higher rate than the general population. Additionally, Vaisman concluded that these problems were caused by the occupational hazard of being chronically exposed to anesthetic gases. Because N_2O was a common denominator in most all anesthetic applications, it was implicated as the causative agent.

B. In the United States Cohen et al[2-4] published articles in the 1970s dealing with anesthetic health hazards. One 1980 published study[5] surveyed more than 50,000 dentists and dental assistants who were exposed to trace anesthetics. The results suggested that long-term exposure to anesthetic gases could be associated with an increase in general health problems and reproductive difficulty. In this study ambient N_2O in the office was not measured and data were collected through memory recall by dental personnel.

C. Since Vaisman's[1] original article the literature has continued to document and describe potential adverse effects of chronic exposure to N_2O. However, this literature has been primarily retrospective in nature; therefore inherent biases in study design were inevitable.[6] Because of these flaws a definitive relationship between the exposure of an individual to N_2O/O_2 and reproductive sequelae cannot be established. Weinberg, Baird, and Rowland[7] addressed these design flaws and proposed recommendations for future studies of this sort.

D. Also during the 1970s Bruce, Bach, and Arbit[8] investigated the possibility of N_2O affecting perceptual cognition and psychomotor skills of personnel exposed to varying concentrations of the gas. Their results were widely noted as they reported audiovisual impairment in just hours of exposure to as little as 50 ppm. Multiple attempts to reproduce the research results of Bruce, Bach, and Arbit[8] have failed; interestingly, these researchers have retracted their conclusions, indicating the results were not based on biologic factors.[9] The National Institute for Occupational Safety and Health (NIOSH) became interested in these and other results being published and in 1977 evaluated the scavenging potential of the equipment used in both the operating room and the outpatient setting. It was determined that 25 ppm was achievable in the operating room but not attainable in a setting such as a dental operatory. Therefore NIOSH chose 50 ppm to be the maximum exposure limit for personnel in a dental setting.[10] Although this limit has not been strictly enforced by the Occupational Safety and Health Administration (OSHA), it remains the recommended standard to date.

E. Despite the negative publicity N_2O received, other studies in the literature claimed no deleterious health effects associated with chronic exposure to N_2O, especially in low concentrations.[11-13] The controversy continued in the literature and was the subject at professional meetings. Both sides of the issue were published; however, because the effects were questionable, the popularity of N_2O/O_2 sedation waned.

F. It became the work of this author to objectively and scientifically evaluate all the published research to verify the possible relationship of chronic exposure to N_2O and its subsequent effects on human health.

   1. In 1995 a worldwide literature search on the topic of biohazards associated with N_2O use was conducted at the University of Colorado. Eight hundred and fifty citations were retrieved, of which 23 met the predetermined criteria for scientific merit.

   2. The conclusions drawn from this literature review clearly indicated that there was no scientific basis for the previously established threshold levels for the hospital operating room or the dental setting.

3. This research became the impetus for a meeting of interested parties representing dentistry, government, and manufacturing. A result of the September 1995 meeting, which was sponsored by the American Dental Association's Council of Scientific Affairs and Council of Dental Practice, was the formal position statement that a maximum N_2O exposure limit in parts per million has not been determined.[14]

II. *Specific Biologic Issues and Health Concerns*

A. Inactivation of methionine synthase was mentioned in Chapter 16. As mentioned, N_2O interferes with this enzyme, which is linked to vitamin B_{12} metabolism. Vitamin B_{12} is necessary for DNA production and subsequent cellular reproduction.

1. Inactivation of methionine synthase occurs rapidly in rats; exposure to 80% N_2O for only 15 minutes revealed inactivation of the enzyme.[15] Because of this interference, it was postulated that fetal development may be impaired because of exposure to N_2O. Animal studies using approximately 60% N_2O for 24 hours on pregnant rats produced miscarriage and other fetal abnormalities.[16]

2. Despite flawed research designs, there has been evidence that chronic exposure to high levels of N_2O does have an effect on reproduction.[5] However, to date there is no evidence that a direct causal relationship exists between reproductive health and scavenged low levels of N_2O.[13,15]

3. Sweeney et al[17] were the first to link reproductive problems in humans with chronic N_2O exposure. He used a sensitive test—the deoxyuridine suppression test—to accurately determine the first signs of this biologic effect in humans.

4. In his research, Sweeney[17] showed that chronic exposure levels of 1800 ppm did not exert any detectable biologic effect. We concur that the level of 400 ppm, as suggested by Sweeney, is a reasonable exposure level that is both attainable and significantly below the biologic threshold established by Sweeney.

5. Because of the significant demands for folic acid during organogenesis (first trimester), postponement of N_2O sedation is recommended. For a pregnant female employed in a setting using N_2O, it is important to know the exposure

levels of N_2O and to use all recommended trace gas scavenging methods. Depending on the individual and the situation, that employee should determine whether she should avoid the office setting and any N_2O exposure for the first trimester.

B. Megaloblastic anemia, first described in the 1950s, was found in patients treated with N_2O for tetanus.[18] Leukopenia and reduced megaloblastic erythropoiesis resembling pernicious anemia ensued.

C. Neurologic disorders associated with chronic N_2O exposure appear as myeloneuropathy. Symptoms such as sensory and proprioception impairment may be permanent but are usually temporary with slow recovery.

III. Current Literature

A. Articles published in the 1990s refer primarily to scavenged vs. unscavenged N_2O levels. In the 1990s practitioners have been educated on ways to effectively scavenge trace gas contamination, with the primary method being the evacuation system and the scavenging nasal hood/mask.

1. The scavenging mask system has become standard for all available designs. When expired N_2O is exhaled through the nose, vacuum suction ports transport this gas through the central suction to the outside atmosphere.

    a. One manufacturer produces a double mask, or a mask within a mask, while others use plastic scavenging cones.

    b. Accutron, Inc. recently introduced a clear, low-profile scavenging cone that attaches to the top of the nasal hood. The transparency of the cone is designed to offer an additional method of monitoring patient respiration.

2. This evacuation flow rate has been established as optimal at 45 lpm.

3. Improved mask designs and/or evacuation devices are being investigated as modifications or additions to the current market.[19-22] As technology advances rapidly, no doubt there will be more efficient products. Ongoing research in this area is encouraged.

B. The published literature has served as a vehicle for informing healthcare professionals of the necessity to analyze N_2O exposure levels in their settings and the ways to minimize trace gas. However, there is evidence that some professionals practice without scavenging equipment and without using any other suggested recommendations.[23-25] Using equipment that does not have scavenging capabilities is clearly a breach of the standard of care.

C. A search of the literature since 1995 uncovered many foreign articles referring to the effectiveness of scavenging trace gas. Several note dramatic decreases in parts per million of N_2O in ambient air when using several scavenging methods.[26-31]

IV. Detection and Monitoring of N_2O

A. Infrared spectrophotometry

1. Infrared spectrophotometry uses radio frequency short electromagnetic energy to detect levels as low as 1 ppm of N_2O in the atmosphere. Figure 17-1 shows an infrared spectrophotometer.

2. Other gases can be detected with this technology as well. An advantage of infrared spectrophotometry is the ability to detect minute levels of gas immediately in the ambient air.

3. The instrument can be rented for a reasonable fee and used to instantly detect the presence of N_2O in any setting.

4. This method of analyzing trace gas contamination in the environment is being recommended to establish a baseline reference of N_2O exposure levels. Depending on the results,

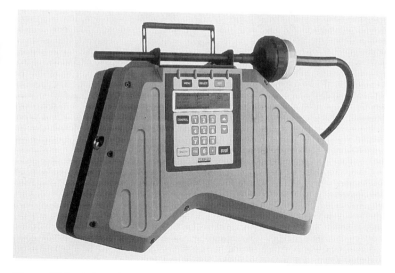

Figure 17-1   Infrared spectrophotometer (Courtesy of Miran, Foxboro Co., East Bridgewater, Mass.).

low levels may be confirmed because of the use of scavenging methods; high levels would indicate the necessity to implement the recommended scavenging methods. Periodic evaluation with this machine is advised.

B. Time-weighted average dosimetry

1. It is also possible to determine the amount of N_2O exposure to an individual over time. This method will give an estimate of the amount of exposure to a gas over a specified period.

2. The badge or vial (similar to a radiation-dosimetry badge) is worn for the recommended period (during exposure or a full work week) and then returned to the company for analysis. An active material in the badge absorbs the N_2O. The amount is read by an infrared spectrophotometer (Figure 17-2) to determine the parts per million of exposure.

3. An advantage to this system is that it is inexpensive and allows for monitoring in a practice not extensively using N_2O. There are several companies that offer these personal monitoring devices. See Appendix A for reference information.

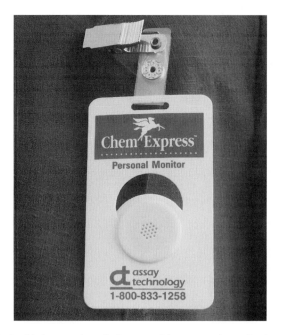

Figure 17-2   Various styles of nitrous oxide personal monitoring devices. (Courtesy of Assay Technology, Palo Alto, Calif; Landauer, Inc, Glenwood, Ill; and Health Career Learning Systems, Inc, Livonia, Mich.)

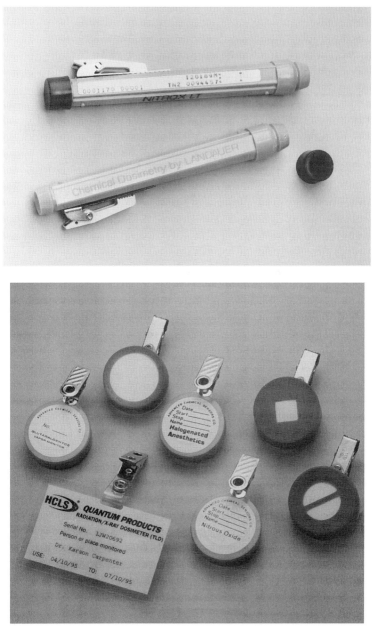

Figure 17-2, cont'd.

V. Scavenging N₂O

A. Scavenging N_2O means minimizing trace amounts of the gas before, during, or after use by the patient.

B. The term *scavenging system* traditionally referred to the mask and suction capabilities of the equipment but is currently a term used to identify several methods for the comprehensive removal of trace N_2O.

C. Certain situations are more problematic for scavenging than others.

    1. Patients that are intubated (i.e., tracheal tube) are in a closed-circuit system that affords every opportunity for complete control over trace waste anesthetic gases.

    2. Patients in an ambulatory setting represent a greater opportunity for trace gas loss because of the open circuitry of the sedation machine. N_2O leakage can be found in several places in this setting (Figure 17-3).

    3. Depending on the location of the office (e.g., in a high-rise building), scavenging efforts may be more difficult with regard to ventilation issues.

D. Sources of leakage from the patient

    1. There are several ways that N_2O can leak from the patient. Perhaps the most critical measure to control in

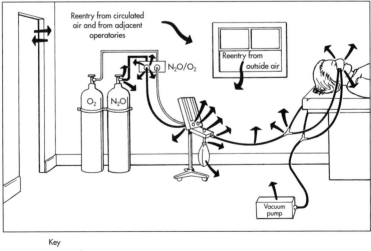

Figure 17-3   Sources of potential N_2O leaks.

this category is patient talking. Whenever the patient talks, he/she is expelling N_2O into the operator's breathing zone. Instruct the patient to breathe through his/her nose and minimize talking.

2. An ill-fitting mask is a potential source for a significant amount of gas leakage. Ensure a snug, comfortable fit and the appropriate tidal volume before titrating N_2O.

3. Other leak sources related to the patient are displacement of the mask during patient movement or restlessness, a technical problem with the mask (e.g., a stuck flutter valve), mouth breathing, or a moustache preventing a tight fit.

E. Sources of leakage other than the patient

1. Gas can leak at any place of connection on the equipment. This includes the manifold and wall-mounted connections and any hoses associated with each.

2. Conducting tubing and the reservoir bag are areas of concern. Because of the breakdown of some materials, it is possible for these items to crack and subsequently leak around pleats and/or seams (Figure 17-4).

3. The soap/water method (Figure 17-5) for determining leaks is recommended for inspecting the areas mentioned in this section. The presence of bubbles after application of the soap/water solution indicates a gas leak.

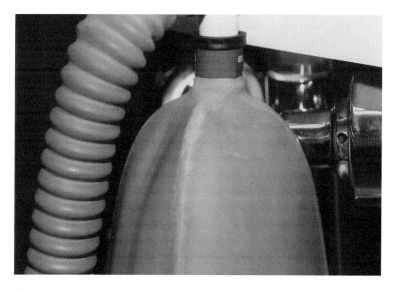

Figure 17-4 N_2O leak potential resulting from breakdown of certain materials.

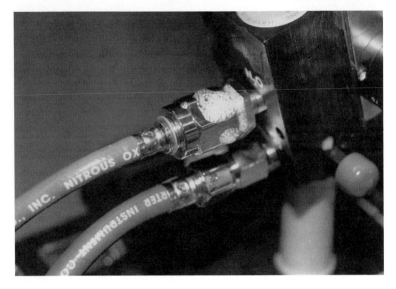

Figure 17-5   Soap/water solution used to test for N$_2$O leaks.

    4. Door seals and any place where reentry of contaminated air could occur is a potential problem.

F. An evacuation (vacuum) system is used to pull trace gas from the mask into the suction for ultimate dispersement to the outside atmosphere.

    1. Again, the optimal flow rate is 45 lpm.

    2. Adjustment of this suction rate is critical for effective sedation. Too much suction will make the gas unavailable for the patient, and not enough suction will create trace gas contamination by leakage around the mask.

    3. It is important to periodically check this flow rate during sedation.

G. Adequate ventilation is an area being investigated for improvement.

    1. In a hospital operating room, fresh-air exchange systems are inherent in the design of the room. In an ambulatory setting such as a dental office there may not be such a provision. Often, air-conditioners recirculate ambient air throughout the office, thereby contributing to contamination rather than N$_2$O elimination. The number of fresh-air exchanges necessary for eliminating trace gas is being investigated.[32]

2. It is recommended that fresh-air inlets be located in the ceiling and designed to direct the fresh-air supply toward the floor to ensure adequate dilution and mixing of the waste gas. Exhaust register louvers should be located near the floor to allow for adequate flushing of the trace N_2O and to prevent short circuiting of the fresh-air supply.[33]

3. Oscillating room fans can be added to assist in moving the gas to a return vent or to an outside source such as an open window.

VI. *Recommendations and Preventive Measures*

A. Monitor the environment for N_2O concentrations.
　1. Establish baseline values if equipment is just being installed. For existing equipment, have the ambient air evaluated periodically using an infrared spectrophotometer.
　2. Monitor the healthcare professional's personal breathing zone (area immediately adjacent to the nose and mouth in a hemisphere forward of the shoulders with a radius of approximately 6 to 9 inches) using time-weighted average dosimetry devices.

B. Prevent leakage from the delivery system through proper maintenance and periodic inspection of the equipment.
　1. Visually inspect the reservoir bag and conduction tubing for cracks and leaks before each administration.
　2. Eliminate or replace loose-fitting connections, loose or deformed slip joints and/or threaded connections, and defective or worn seals or gaskets.
　3. Periodically send the sedation equipment back to the manufacturer (depending on their recommendation) for routine evaluation and maintenance. Do not alter, modify, or attempt to adjust this equipment.

C. Control waste N_2O with an appropriate evacuation system that includes securely fitting masks, sufficient evacuation flow rates (45 lpm), and properly vented pumps.

D. Assess the adequacy of room ventilation and air exchange for effectively removing waste N_2O.
　1. If concentrations are above 25 ppm but less than 150 ppm, it is recommended to increase exhausting capabilities in the area.[34]
　2. Supplement local ventilation to capture the N_2O at the source, add oscillating sweep fans, and/or increase the airflow and air exchange to the room.

E. Institute an educational program for members of the health-care team, which describes the hazards of N_2O and defines the prevention measures for reducing/eliminating trace gas contamination.

VII. *Summary*

A. N_2O/O_2 sedation is a very valuable tool in the ambulatory health setting for the control of pain and anxiety. We will continue to rely on its effectiveness.

B. To date there is no direct evidence of any causal relationship between chronic low-level exposure to N_2O and potential biologic effects. The maximum safe concentration of N_2O has not been determined; however, every attempt should be made to reduce the level of trace N_2O to exposed healthcare personnel. We cannot be too cautious when the health of ourselves and coworkers is at stake.

C. Continued research efforts for the scientific advancement of topics related to chronic exposure of N_2O and additional ways to minimize and/or eliminate trace gas contamination are encouraged. Emphasis should be placed on prospective and well-designed studies. Manufacturers should be encouraged to continue their efforts at creating and maintaining effective and efficient equipment.

D. Continuing education should be required of healthcare professionals using N_2O/O_2 sedation, as should evidence of proper training using state-of-the-art equipment and administration techniques.

REFERENCES

1. Vaisman A: Working conditions in surgery and their effect on the health of anesthesiologists, *Eksp Khir Anesteziol* 3:44-49, 1967.
2. Cohen EN, Belville JW, Brown BW: Anesthesia, pregnancy and miscarriage: a study of operating room nurses and anesthetists, *Anesthesiology* 35:343-347, 1971.
3. Cohen EN et al: Occupational disease among operating room personnel: a national study, *Anesthesiology* 41:321-340, 1974.
4. Cohen EN et al: A survey of anesthetic health hazards among dentists: report of an American Society of Anesthesiologists ad hoc committee on the effects of trace anesthetics on the health of operating room personnel, *J Am Dent Assoc* 90:1291-1296, 1975.
5. Cohen EN et al: Occupational disease in dentistry and chronic exposure to trace anesthetic gases, *J Am Dent Assoc* 101:21-31, 1980.
6. Clark MS, Renehan BW, Jeffers BW: Clinical use and potential biohazards of nitrous oxide/oxygen, *Gen Dent* 45:486-491, 1997.

7. Weinberg CR, Baird DD, Rowland AS: Pitfalls inherent in retrospective time-to-event studies: the example of time to pregnancy, *Stat Med* 12:867-879, 1993.

8. Bruce DL, Bach MJ, Arbit J: Trace anesthetic effects on perceptual, cognitive, and motor skills, *Anesthesiology* 40:453-458, 1974.

9. Yagiela JA: Health hazards and nitrous oxide: a time for reappraisal, *Anesth Prog* 38:1-11, 1991.

10. Bruce DL, Bach MJ: Trace effects of anesthetic gases on behavioral performance of operating room personnel, HEW publication No (NIOSH) 76-169, Cincinnati, 1976, US Department of Health, Education, and Welfare.

11. Ericson HA, Kallen AB: Hospitalization for miscarriage and delivery outcome among Swedish nurses working in operating rooms in 1973-1978, *Anest Anal* 64:981-988, 1985.

12. Hemminke K, Kyyronen P, Lindbohm ML: Spontaneous abortions and malformation in the offspring of nurses exposed to anaesthetic gases, cytostatic drugs, and other potential hazards in hospitals based on registered information of outcome, *J Epidemiol Community Health* 39:141-147, 1985.

13. Rowland AS et al: Reduced fertility among women employed as dental assistants exposed to high levels of nitrous oxide, *New Eng J Med* 327:993-997, 1992.

14. ADA Council on Scientific Affairs, ADA Council on Dental Practice: Nitrous oxide in the dental office, *J Am Dent Assoc* 128:364-365, 1997.

15. Eger II EI: Fetal injury and abortion associated with occupational exposure to inhaled anesthetics, *J Am Assoc Nurse Anesth* 59:309-312, 1991.

16. Fujinagra M, Baden JM, Mazze RI: Susceptible period of nitrous oxide teratogenicity in Sprague-Dawley rats, *Teratology* 40:439-444, 1989.

17. Sweeney B et al: Toxicity of bone marrow in dentists exposed to nitrous oxide, *Br Med J* 291:567-569, 1985.

18. Lassen JA et al: Treatment of tetanus: severe bone-marrow depression after prolonged nitrous-oxide anaesthesia, *Lancet* 1:527-530, 1956.

19. Crouch KG, Johnston OE: Nitrous oxide control in the dental operatory: auxiliary exhaust and mask leakage, design, and scavenging flow rate as factors, *Am Ind Hyg Assoc J* 57:272-278, 1996.

20. Donaldson D, Grabi J: The efficiency of nitrous oxide scavenging devices in dental offices, *J Can Dent Assoc* 55:541-543, 1989.

21. Ooi R, Joshi P, Soni N: Nitrous oxide/oxygen analgesia: the performance of the MC mask delivery system, *J Royal Soc Med* 85:534-536, 1992.

22. Shafer SM: Face mask scavenging system, *J Oral Maxillofac Surg* 51:945-946, 1993.

23. Dunning DG, McFarland K, Safarik M: Nitrous-oxide use. I. Risk of potential exposure and compliance among Nebraska dentists and dental assistants, *Gen Dent* 44:520-523, 1997.

24. Wilson S: A survey of the American Academy of Pediatric Dentistry membership: nitrous oxide and sedation, *Pediatr Dent* 18:287-293, 1996.

25. ECRI Reporting System: Hazard update: nitrous oxide cryosurgical units must be scavenged, *Health Devices* 25:306-309, 1996.

26. Schuyt HC, Verberk MM: Measurement and reduction of nitrous oxide in operating rooms, *Occup Environ Med* 38:1036-1040, 1996.

27. Imberti R, Preseglio I, Imbriani M: Low flow anaesthesia reduces occupational exposure to inhalation anaesthetics, *Acta Anaes Scand* 39:586-591, 1995.

28. Lucchini R, Toffoletto F, Camerino D: Neurobehavioral functions in operating theatre personnel exposed to anesthetic gases, *Med Lav* 86:27-33, 1995.

29. Hoerauf KH et al: Occupational exposure to sevoflurane and nitrous oxide in operating room personnel, *Int Arch Occup Environ Health* 69:134-138, 1997.

30. Chang WP, Kau CW, Hseu SS: Exposure of anesthesiologists to nitrous oxide during pediatric anesthesia, *Ind Health* 35:112-118, 1997.
31. Ahlborg Jr G, Axelsson G, Bodin L: Shift work, nitrous oxide exposure and sub-fertility among Swedish midwives, *Int J Epidemiol* 25:783-790, 1996.
32. Borganelli GN, Primosch RE, Henry RJ: Operatory ventilation and scavenger evacuation rate influence on ambient nitrous oxide levels, *J Dent Res* 72:1275-1278, 1993.
33. Howard WR: Nitrous oxide in the dental environment: assessing the risk, reducing the exposure, *J Am Dent Assoc* 128:356-360, 1997.
34. McGlothlin JD, Crouch KG, Mickelsen RI: Control of nitrous oxide in dental operatories, DHHS No (NIOSH) 94-129, Cincinnati, 1994, US Department of Health and Human Services, Public Health Service, Centers for Disease Control and Prevention, National Institute for Occupational Safety and Health, Division of Physical Sciences and Engineering, Engineering Control Technology Branch.

SUGGESTED READINGS

There are many published articles that address this topic. Those listed in the references are a select few. This is not a complete bibliography.

18

Ethical and Legal Concerns Regarding Nitrous Oxide Administration

Has today's litigious society created bitter, callous healthcare professionals? Has the high moral standard of yesterday diminished such that a conscience need not exist? Where does the line cross over to greed? Is practicing healthcare today worth the legal and ethical hassles?

I. Appropriate Education for N_2O/O_2 Administration

A. Depending on the discipline and the governing body regulating the parameters of practice within the discipline, there may be rules to abide by regarding the administration of N_2O/O_2 sedation.

1. There are widespread variations among disciplines as to who may administer and/or monitor the N_2O/O_2 sedation procedure; the profession determines who is or is not eligible to provide this type of service and under what conditions it may be administered. These parameters of practice are monitored by the appropriate governing agency, whose purpose is to protect the public.

   a. Depending on the discipline, a practitioner may only be legally allowed to monitor a patient under N_2O/O_2 sedation and not be allowed to administer the drug. This would prohibit the individual from titrating N_2O to the patient. This may be the case for certain levels of auxiliaries within a discipline.

   b. Because there are so many legal variations of rules that are discipline specific, it is critical to be informed of the codified law and administrative rules applicable to each discipline.

2. Governing boards/licensing agencies may require a specified course of training in the area of N_2O/O_2 sedation

before practitioners can incorporate this procedure into their clinical practices.

    a. Often, proof of successful completion of a previously approved course on the subject is required. Approved courses usually consist of both didactic and clinical components, totaling a specified minimum number of hours.

    b. After successful completion of such a course of study and probable fee payment, the practitioner may be granted a permit or license to administer N_2O/O_2 sedation.

    c. Most often, students completing their professional curriculum are exempt from additional coursework in this area unless this information was not part of the professional program. In such a case the student would be subject to the same requirements as those without the necessary education.

B. It may be favorable for a previously educated practitioner to participate in a N_2O/O_2 sedation refresher course. Updated material, new equipment, or a review of the appropriate administration technique may be presented, which could enhance the success of this procedure in clinical practice. The authors have found that those participating in review courses return to their practices with a renewed appreciation for the drug and its potential. They value the reinforcement of how the procedure is making their practice successful while providing a valuable service to their patients.

II. Prudent Practice Guidelines

A. The propensity exists for a patient to become sexually stimulated or dream/hallucinate sexual situations while sedated with N_2O. There are obvious ways to avoid allegations of sexual misconduct. Common sense is all that is necessary in most cases.

    1. Use the appropriate technique and titrate to the exact level of appropriate sedation. Most patients will achieve this endpoint at N_2O concentrations less than 50%. If the patient requires a percentage higher than 50%, the operator should be alert that cumulative effects of the drug may quickly change the level of sedation and that this range is considered high risk for dreaming or fantasizing.

    2. Have a third party in the room during the procedure as a witness against false accusations. If a third-party witness

is not feasible, it is recommended to alert a fellow professional that concentrations of near 50% are being administered and to be available for frequent checking in on the procedure.

3. Do not place yourself in a potentially incriminating situation, such as an after-hours appointment where intentions may be misinterpreted.

B. Be meticulous about record keeping and documentation procedures. Record the details of each sedation experience for every patient in the treatment file.

C. Practice within the standard of care established by the profession. Use updated equipment with the O_2 fail-safe mechanism for safe delivery to the patient. Follow the steps for appropriate N_2O/O_2 administration. Use the recommended scavenging procedures for the sake of those exposed to trace gas contamination.

D. Maintain an adequate and current malpractice insurance policy.

E. Practice within the parameters of the discipline. Do not ask others to perform the procedure when they are not legally allowed to do so, or do not perform the task yourself if you are not permitted.

III. *Ethical Responsibilities*

A. In addition to legal practice guidelines for administering N_2O/O_2 sedation, there are ethical aspects to consider. N_2O/O_2 sedation is available for reducing a patient's pain and anxiety before performing a clinical procedure. It would be unethical for a healthcare professional to knowingly administer N_2O to a patient for any other reason (e.g., thrill seeking).

B. The abuse potential of N_2O has been discussed (see Chapter 16). It is the responsibility of the practitioner to ensure that tanks are properly stored and locked securely so that the likelihood of others stealing a tank or abusing N_2O is minimized.

C. Do not abuse N_2O yourself. There are significant health risks and complications that could affect you permanently. Seek help if necessary.

D. Use updated, state-of-the-art equipment provided by the manufacturers. The delivery systems currently available undergo stringent, quality control and safety measures. Use the recommended scavenging techniques and procedures for minimizing trace gas contamination to exposed personnel.

19

Future Trends in Nitrous Oxide/Oxygen Sedation

Unquestionably, as we enter the new millenium, change will occur. It will be a new era, a new beginning; many aspects of life will not be the same. There are those of us who will watch and wait and follow, and there will be those of us who will walk boldly and lead. There is no doubt that there will be governmental influence in healthcare. Bureaucracy will be our partner whether invited or not. We will survive and we will thrive. Our contentment will depend on the things that satisfy us. It is hoped that the inner desire to improve our neighbor's health stands out in the forefront.

It is our duty to become involved with those agencies and individuals who are responsible for safe products and safe procedures. We have faith that the manufacturers of nitrous oxide/oxygen (N_2O/O_2) equipment will continue to provide you and the patient with the highest quality products available and will pursue technologic avenues for minimizing trace gas contamination. There is no doubt that the industry will continue its dedication to providing quality equipment for the safe delivery of N_2O and O_2.

The delivery of inhalation sedation using N_2O/O_2 is being enhanced in many ways. An example of modern day use can be seen in the Flying Hospital, a fully equipped, airborne surgical facility. Figure 19-1 shows the layout of the Flying Hospital.

Several disciplines are already broadening their scope of practice to allow additional professionals to administer N_2O/O_2 sedation. If the trend continues to focus on ambulatory healthcare, there will be a need for additional personnel in the field to deliver this service.

Market predictions indicate an increase in the consumption of N_2O. Patients will continue to undergo surgical procedures at an increasing rate. Populations are growing older; healthcare will always be a priority. N_2O/O_2 sedation will be a useful part of the future. It can be of great assistance to you.

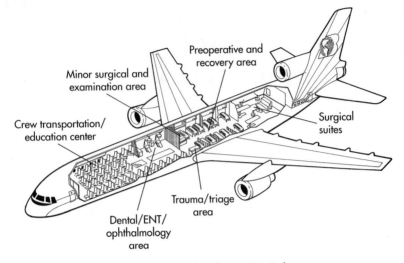

Figure 19-1 The Flying Hospital.

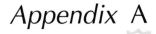

Appendix A

Address List for Manufacturers and Organizational Resources

Authors

Clark, Morris DDS, FACD
Department of Oral and Maxillofacial Surgery
University of Colorado Health Sciences Center
4200 East 9th Street
Denver, CO 80262
Phone: 303-315-6345
Fax: 303-315-0336

Brunick, Ann RDH, MS
Department of Dental Hygiene, 120 East Hall
University of South Dakota
414 East Clark Street
Vermillion, SD 57069
Phone: 605-677-5379
Fax: 605-677-5638

Nitrous Oxide/Oxygen Equipment Manufacturers

Accutron, Inc.
2020 West Melinda Lane
Phoenix, AZ 85027
Phone: 800-531-2221
Fax: 602-780-0444

MDS Matrx Medical Inc.
145 Med County Drive
Orchard Park, NY 14127
Phone: 800-847-1000
Fax: 716-662-7130
matrxmedical.com

Porter Instrument Co., Inc.
245 Township Line Road, Box 907
Hatfield, PA 19440-0907
Phone: 800-457-2001
Fax: 215-723-2199
porterinst.com

Personal Monitoring Devices

Advanced Chemical Sensor, Inc.
3201 North Dixie Highway
Boca Raton, FL 33431
Phone: 561-338-3116
Fax: 561-338-5737

Assay Technology
1070 East Meadow Circle
Palo Alto, CA 94303-4230
Phone: 800-833-1258
assaytec.com

Health Career Learning Systems, Inc.
37557 Schoolcraft Road
Livonia, MI 48150
Phone: 800-829-4257
hclsinc.com

Kem Medical Products Corp.
14 Engineers Lane
Farmingdale, NY 11735
Phone: 800-553-0330
Fax: 516-454-8083
kemmed.com

Landauer, Inc.
2 Science Road
Glenwood, IL 60425-1586
Phone: 708-755-7000
Fax: 708-755-7016
landauerinc.com

Nevin Laboratories, Inc.
5000 South Halsted Street
Chicago, IL 60609
Phone: 800-544-5337

Infrared Spectrophotometry

The Foxboro Co.
600 North Bedford Street, Box 500
East Bridgewater, MA 02333
Phone: 800-321-0322
Fax: 508-378-5505
foxboro.com

Organizational Resources

American Conference of Government Industrial Hygienists
1330 Keniper Meadow Drive, Suite 600
Cincinnati, OH 45240
Phone: 513-742-2020
Fax: 513-742-3355

American Dental Association
211 East Chicago Avenue
Chicago, IL 60611
Phone: 800-621-8099
Fax: 312-440-7494
ada.org

American Dental Hygienists' Association
444 North Michigan Avenue, Suite 3400
Chicago, IL 60611
Phone: 312-440-8900
Fax: 312-440-8929
adha.org

American Dental Society of Anesthesiology
211 East Chicago Avenue, Suite 780
Chicago, IL 60611
Phone: 800-722-7788
Fax: 312-642-9713
adsahome.org

American Medical Association
515 North State Street
Chicago, IL 60611
Phone: 312-464-5000
Fax: 312-464-4184
ama-assn.org

American Society of Anesthesiologists
520 North Northwest Highway
Park Ridge, IL 60068-2573
Phone: 847-825-5586
Fax: 847-825-1692
asahq.org

Centers for Disease Control (CDC)
1600 Clifton Road NE
Atlanta, GA 30333
Phone: 404-639-3311
cdc.gov

Compressed Gas Association, Inc.
1725 Jefferson Davis Highway, Suite 1004
Arlington, VA 22202-4102
Phone: 703-412-0900
Fax: 703-412-0128
cganet.com

Piping, Industry, Progress, and Education (P.I.P.E.)
501 Shatto Place, Suite 200
Los Angeles, CA 90020
Phone: 800-457-7473
Fax: 213-382-2501
pipe.org

National Fire Protection Association
1 Batterymarch Park, Box 9101
Quincy, MA 02269-9101
Phone: 617-770-3000
Fax: 617-770-0700
nfpa.org

National Institute for Occupational Safety and Health (NIOSH)
4676 Columbia Parkway
Cincinnati, OH 45226
Phone: 800-356-4674
Fax: 513-533-8573
cdc.gov/niosh

National Inspection Testing Certification (ITC)
Ron Ridenour
Executive Director
501 Shatto Place
Suite 200
Los Angeles, CA 90020
Phone: 213-382-5255

National Welding Supply Association
1900 Arch Street
Philadelphia, PA 19103
Phone: 215-564-3484
Fax: 215-564-2175
nwsa.com

Nellcor Puritan Bennett Inc.
9101 Bond Street
Overland Park, KS 66214
Phone: 913-495-3606
Fax: 913-495-3698
nellcorpb.com

Occupational Safety and Health Administration (OSHA)
Health Standards Programs
United States Department of Labor
200 Constitution Avenue NW
Washington, DC 20210
Phone: 202-219-7075
osha.gov

TABLE B-1
N_2O/O_2 Percentage Chart

Liters Per Minute N_2O	Liters Per Minute O_2									
	1	2	3	4	5	6	7	8	9	10
1	50	33	25	20	17	14	13	11	10	9
2	67	50	40	33	29	25	22	20	18	17
3	75*	60	50	43	38	33	30	27	25	23
4	80*	67	57	50	44	40	36	33	31	29
5	83*	71	63	56	50	45	42	38	36	33
6	86*	75*	67	60	55	50	46	43	40	38
7	88*	78*	70	64	58	54	50	46	44	41
8	89*	80*	73	67	62	57	53	50	47	44
9	90*	82*	75*	69	64	60	56	53	50	47
10	91*	83*	77*	71	67	63	59	56	53	50

*Percentage exceeds maximum amount of N_2O needed for effective pain/anxiety management in an ambulatory setting and exceeds amounts able to be delivered by analgesia machines.

TABLE C-1
N_2O/O_2 Percentage Chart for Constant O_2 Flow Technique: 7.0 L/min O_2

N_2O L/min	O_2	% N_2O
0	7.0	0
1	7.0	13
2	7.0	22
3	7.0	30
4	7.0	36
5	7.0	42
6	7.0	46
7	7.0	50

TABLE C-2
N_2O/O_2 Percentage Chart for Constant O_2 Flow Technique: 6.0 L/min O_2

N_2O L/min	O_2	% N_2O
0	6.0	0
1	6.0	14
2	6.0	25
3	6.0	33
4	6.0	40
5	6.0	45
6	6.0	50

TABLE C-3
N_2O/O_2 Percentage Chart for Constant O_2 Flow Technique: 5.0 L/min O_2

N_2O L/min	O_2	% N_2O
1	5.0	17
2	5.0	29
3	5.0	38
4	5.0	44
5	5.0	50

N₂O/O₂
Sedation Record

Date: _____ Patient: _____ Age: ____

ASA classification: I   II   III   IV

Med consult needed: Yes/No   Operative procedure: _____

Procedural data:

	PREOPERATIVE		POSTOPERATIVE
BP:	_____		_____
Pulse/Quality:	_____		_____
Respiration:	_____		_____

N_2O Start time: _____ N_2O Finish time: _____

Titrated % of N_2O: _____   Postoperative O_2: _____
  (for documentation purposes only)   (in minutes)

Comments:

Clinician signature: _____

Appendix E

Administration of N_2O/O_2 Sedation

1. Inspect all N_2O/O_2 equipment for proper setup. Periodically check pressure connections with a soap/water solution as per manufacturer's recommendations. Inspect the tubing and reservoir bag for cracks or tears.

2. Confirm the adequacy of all scavenging methods to include the vacuum exhaust and ventilation for the area.

3. Review the patient's health history and record vital signs. Obtain informed consent.

4. Activate O_2 flow, fit nasal hood/face mask, and establish appropriate tidal volume. Observe reservoir bag.

5. Initiate N_2O flow and titrate appropriately while constantly assessing the patient.

6. Upon termination of the N_2O, begin a minimum postoxygenation period of 3 to 5 minutes.

7. Assess the patient for appropriate recovery. Administer additional O_2 if necessary.

8. Document the procedure appropriately in the patient's file (i.e., sedation record).

9. Properly disassemble and disinfect equipment.

Index

Page numbers in italics indicate illustrations.
Page numbers followed by a *b* indicate boxes.
Page numbers followed by *t* indicate tables.